Thanks to
Bret Frey, M.D.

# INTRODUCTION

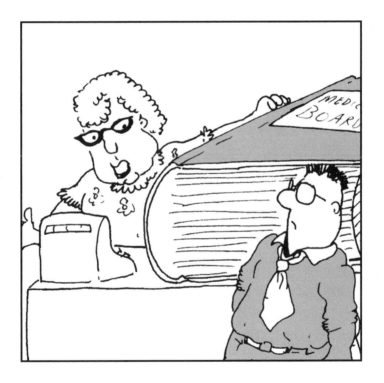

"This is the most complete book for the USMLE.
It even has clinically relevant material."

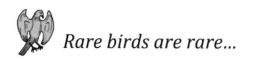
*Rare birds are rare...*

# PREFACE TO THE 4<sup>th</sup> EDITION

The USMLE Step 3 has changed significantly since I wrote the 1<sup>st</sup> edition of this book and has become more difficult than it used to be. You cannot rely on simple "high-yield-facts" anymore and a thorough understanding of patient management and prioritization is most important. Computer-based case simulations now account for about 25% of your score. I have completely rewritten this book for the new USMLE Step 3 format and the old chapter 2 (Preventive Medicine and Epidemiology) has been replaced with **Patient Management.** A brief overview chapter about health prevention, cancer screening and immunization schedules has been added. Most information is presented in a simple step-by-step approach. All treatment recommendations have been carefully brought up-to-date.

I wish to thank the many students whose input has allowed me to keep this book current and relevant for the USMLE exam.

Please visit my web-site to share your experiences with other students:

## www.usmle.net

If you are about to take the exam or just took it, you can contact me via e-mail:

## andreas_carl@usmle.net

## USMLE STEP 3 FORMAT

Compared to the Step 2 exam, questions tend to be more complex, more information is presented and it will take longer to read through the cases. I always recommend to read the last sentence of each case presentation, to get an idea what the question is about. This way you can read more selectively and extract the useful information.

All questions are single best choice and arranged in settings:

- Satellite Health Center
- Office
- Hospital
- Emergency Department.

While this format is intended to make the exam more "realistic" you will find that it has surprisingly little effect on your actual test taking. You still will have to answer each question based solely on the information presented in each case.

Many questions on the USMLE Step 3 exam end with a phrase like "the most appropriate next step would be to...", "the most appropriate intervention would be..." and similar expressions. *USMLE Step 3 Made Ridiculously Simple* gives you information in a step-by-step fashion to help you answer exactly this type of questions.

## WHICH BOOK SHOULD I USE?

You should use the same materials you already used for your Step 2 preparation since you are familiar with these and it makes for the most efficient review. If you have used my *USMLE Step 2 Made Ridiculously Simple* book - great! I strongly recommend you take a day or two and go over the charts presented there. About 10% of the questions on the Step 3 exam are Basic Science and it is important to review the Pharmacology and Pathology chapters from my Step 1 book. For additional updated information about popular study aids, please visit my website.

### WHAT IS THE DIFFERENCE BETWEEN THIS STEP 3 AND MY STEP 2 BOOK?

*USMLE Step 3 Made Ridiculously Simple* is the perfect companion to my *USMLE Step 2 Made Ridiculously Simple* book. While the Step 2 book presents material in a "disease-oriented approach" centered around organ systems, the Step 3 book presents material in a more "patient-oriented approach".

The two books are designed to go "hand-in-hand" and complement each other. The Step 2 book will give you a solid foundation to pass the Step 2 exam and also would serve you well for the Step 3. My *USMLE Step 3 Made Ridiculously Simple* extends the material into areas which are emphasized on the USMLE Step 3 exam, namely diagnostic approaches and patient management. You can use *USMLE Step 3 Made Ridiculously Simple* together with my Step 2 book or to supplement other review books you like to use.

All areas of Medicine are covered in both books, however the emphasis is different:

| STEP 2 book | STEP 3 book |
|---|---|
| • Diseases and Organ Systems | • Diagnosis, Step-by-Step<br>• Patient Management |

## IMPORTANT DISCLAIMER:

The diagnostic and therapeutic algorithms in this book are meant as examples only and not for treatment of actual patients. Real-world medicine is more complicated than what can be presented in a book like this. The purpose of these diagnostic and therapeutic algorithms is to remind you of common approaches to typical medical problems you may encounter on the USMLE Step 3 exam. When treating a patient, you will often deviate from any such schematics, depending on each individual case. Always treat the patient, not the symptoms!

Numbers given about prevalence and prognosis do NOT need to be memorized for the exam. They are meant only to give the student a rough idea about the outcome and how likely to encounter them in "real life". Remember, rare birds are rare – but not on the USMLE.

## HOW TO USE THIS BOOK?

**Chapter 1** gives a very brief overview about preventive medicine, cancer screening and immunization schedules. These are very important to memorize. Also a brief list of "ethical dilemmas" you will encounter in exam questions. These are important!

**Chapter 2** presents a **step-by-step** approach to medical diagnosis, beginning with a symptom or sign followed by diagnostic tests arranged systematically from top to bottom in flow-charts. The diagnostic tests presented at the top of each charts are the least invasive and typically give the highest yield.
The tests at the bottom of each chart are the most invasive with the lowest yield. You should pay careful attention to the order of these tests. It is assumed that you work your way from top to bottom, proceeding to the next test, if the results from the previous one were negative.

**Chapter 3** presents patient management in a similar **step-by-step** fashion. You need to know about risk factors and prevention of disease and simple treatment algorithms. Please keep in mind that *USMLE Step 3 Made Ridiculously Simple* is not a textbook but a supplement. Facts are presented in a logical and easily accessible format in order to help you review the key info just prior to the exam.

Chapters 2 and 3 are arranged in alphabetical fashion for easy reference. For students and residents who have the time and wish to prepare themselves in a more systematic way, a **Table of Contents by Organ Systems** is provided. It is hoped that this book will not only be useful for your exam preparation but also as a quick refresher course during your clinical years. How you score on the USMLE Step 3 exam not only depends on how hard you study, but also on what you study. Obviously, if you study what they ask, you will achieve a very high score. Care has been taken not to overload this book with "rare birds"...

> ➢ Use it during your clinical work to organize your thoughts
> ➢ Use it as a refresher course
> ➢ Use it as a last minute review

You can – and should !!! – use this book as a TESTING TOOL in a similar fashion like you would study vocabulary of a foreign language: Cover the right part of the chart with your hand, and check if you can recall the key features or key associations of each item:

## 1.3.) PREGNANCY SCREENING

| hypertension | • monitor throughout pregnancy (weight gain, edema, blood pressure) |
|---|---|
| Rh incompatibility | • determine at first prenatal visit |
| rubella titer | • determine at first prenatal visit |
| STDS | screen at first prenatal visit: norrhea |
| bacteriuria | • ___ prenatal visit<br>• ___ if asymptomatic |
| triple screen [1] | • at 16 |
| oral glucose tolerance | • at 24~28 week |
| amniocentesis | • consider for w |

*"Praying hands" borrowed from Albrecht Dürer.*

I wish to thank Steve Goldberg for the cartoons. I hope that this text will help your preparation for the USMLE Step 3 and would appreciate any comments about the selection and presentation of this material you might have. Good luck!

# www.usmle.net
➢ latest trends on the USMLE
➢ discussion forums
➢ book recommendations

ෲෲෲෲෲෲෲෲෲෲෲෲෲෲෲෲ

## REFERENCES

1. Cecil Textbook of Medicine, W.B. Saunders Co.
2. Current Medical Diagnosis&Treatment, Appleton&Lange
3. Current Emergency Diagnosis&Treatment, Appleton&Lange
4. Current Obstetric&Gynecologic Diagnosis&Treatment, Appleton&Lange
5. Current Pediatric Diagnosis&Treatment, Appleton&Lange
6. Decision Making in Medicine, Mosby
7. Dermatology in General Medicine, McGraw-Hill
8. Harrison's Principles of Internal Medicine, McGraw-Hill
9. Heart Disease - A Textbook of Cardiovascular Medicine, W.B. Saunders Co.
10. Internal Medicine, Ed. J.H. Stein, Mosby
11. Mayo Internal Medicine Board Review, Mayo Foundation
12. Obstetrics and Gynecology, J.B. Lippincott Co.
13. Principles and Practice of Infectious Diseases, Churchill Livingstone
14. Principles of Neurology, McGraw-Hill
15. Rudolph's Pediatrics, Appleton&Lange
16. Synopsis of Psychiatry, Williams&Wilkins
17. Williams Hematology, McGraw-Hill

ෲෲෲෲෲෲෲෲෲෲෲෲෲෲෲෲ

## INTERNATIONAL MEDICAL GRADUATES

It is highly recommended for IMGs to take the Step 3 exam **BEFORE** applying for residency training; this way you are eligible for an H1-B visa. Without Step 3 you can get only a temporary J1 visa.

# CONTENTS

# TABLE OF CONTENTS BY ORGAN SYSTEMS

## RESPIRATORY DISEASES

| | | | |
|---|---|---|---|
| 2.5. | Acidosis | 2.55. | Hemoptysis |
| 2.9. | Alkalosis | 2.59. | Hypercapnia |
| 3.8. | Altitude sickness | 3.140. | Influenza |
| 3.20. | ARDS | 3.152. | Legionnaires' disease |
| 3.23. | Asthma | 3.157. | Lung cancer |
| 3.24. | Atelectasis | 2.86. | Pleural effusion |
| 3.40. | Bronchiectasis | 3.202. | Pneumonia - bacterial |
| 3.41. | Bronchiolitis | 3.203. | Pneumonia - mycoplasma |
| 2.28. | Chest pain | 3.204. | Pneumonia - PCP |
| 3.63. | COPD | 3.205. | Pneumonia - viral |
| 3.65. | Cor pulmonale | 3.232. | Sarcoidosis |
| 2.30. | Cough | 3.239. | Silicosis |
| 2.31. | Cyanosis | 2.99. | Stridor - children |
| 3.71. | Cystic fibrosis | 2.100. | Stridor - adults |
| 2.39. | Dyspnea | 3.264. | Tuberculosis |

## GASTROINTESTINAL DISEASES

| | | | |
|---|---|---|---|
| 2.1. | Acute abdomen | 3.110 | Gastroesophageal reflux disease |
| 2.2. | Abdominal pain - upper | | |
| 2.3. | Abd. Pain - periumbilical | 2.49. | GI bleeding |
| 2.4. | Abdominal pain - lower | 3.111. | Giardiasis |
| 2.8. | Alkaline phosphatase | 3.119. | Hemochromatosis |
| 2.22. | Ascites | 3.121. | Hepatitis |
| 3.47. | Celiac disease | 3.122 | Hepatocellular adenoma |
| 3.53. | Cholecystitis | 3.123. | Hepatocellular carcinoma |
| 3.54. | Cholelithiasis | 2.56. | Hepatomegaly |
| 3.60. | Colorectal cancer | 3.142. | Intestinal obstruction |
| 2.29. | Constipation | 3.143. | Intussusception |
| 3.61. | Constipation | 3.144. | Irritable bowel syndrome |
| 3.66. | Crohn's disease | 2.73. | Jaundice |
| 2.33. | Diarrhea - acute | 3.150. | Lactose intolerance |
| 2.34. | Diarrhea - chronic | 3.156. | Liver cirrhosis |
| 3.82. | Diverticulosis | 3.191. | Pancreas cancer |
| 3.86. | Dyspepsia | 3.192. | Pancreatitis |
| 2.38. | Dysphagia | 3.195. | Peptic ulcer disease |
| 3.99. | Esophageal cancer | 3.214. | Pseudomembranous colitis |
| 3.103. | Food allergy | 3.220. | Pyloric stenosis |
| 3.106. | Gastric adenocarcinoma | 2.108. | Transaminases |
| 3.107. | Gastritis, chronic type A | 3.269. | Ulcerative colitis |
| 3.108 | Gastritis, chronic type B | 3.278. | Zollinger-Ellison syndrome |
| 3.109 | Gastritis, erosive | | |

## UROGENITAL DISEASES / STDS

## HEMATOLOGICAL DISEASES

# ENDOCRINE DISEASES

3.6. Addison's disease
3.7. Aldosteronism
3.69. Cushing's syndrome
3.74. Diabetes mellitus type 1
3.75. Diabetes mellitus type 2
3.76. Diabetic hypoglycemia
3.77. Diabetic ketoacidosis
3.78. Diabetic retinopathy

2.50. Gynecomastia
2.61. Hyperlipidemia
2.66. Hypoglycemia
3.199. Pheochromocytoma
3.255. Thyroid cancer
2.105. Thyroid enlargement
2.106. Thyroid nodule

# MUSCULOSKELETAL DISEASES

2.8. Alkaline phosphatase
3.13. Ankylosing spondylitis
2.21. Arthralgia
3.115. Gout
3.127. Hip fracture
3.138. Infectious arthritis
3.146. Juvenile idiopathic arthritis
2.74. Lower back pain
3.162. Marfan's syndrome
2.80. Muscle weakness
3.176. Muscular dystrophy
3.177. Myasthenia gravis

3.185. Osgood Schlatter disease
3.186. Osteoarthritis
3.187. Osteomyelitis
3.188. Osteoporosis
3.210. Polymyositis / Dermatomyositis
3.222. Raynaud's phenomenon
3.223. Reiter's syndrome
3.228. Rheumatoid arthritis
3.249. SLE
3.251. Temporomandibular joint syndrome

# DISEASES OF THE EYE AND SKIN

3.3. Acne vulgaris
3.4. Actinic keratosis
2.10. Alopecia
3.14. Anorectal abscess
3.25. Atopic dermatitis
3.32. Basal cell carcinoma
3.62. Contact dermatitis
3.70. Cutaneous drug reactions
3.80. Discoid lupus erythematosus
3.96. Erysipelas
3.105. Gangrene
3.112. Glaucoma
3.126. Herpes zoster
2.57. Hirsutism
3.147. Kaposi sarcoma
3.148. Keloids
3.164. Melanoma
3.184. Onychomycosis

3.211. Porphyria
2.91. Pruritus
3.216. Psoriasis
2.92. Purpura
2.44. Red eye
2.113. Retina
3.225. Retinal detachment
3.226. Retrolental fibroplasia
3.235. Seborrhoic dermatitis
2.96. Skin rash - adults
2.97. Skin rash - children
3.241. Squamous cell carcinoma
3.242. Stasis dermatitis / ulcer
2.110. Urticaria
3.275. Vitiligo
2.113. Vision loss
3.276. Warts

## OBSTETRICS & GYNECOLOGY

## PEDIATRIC DISEASES

# INFECTIOUS DISEASES

# MALIGNANCIES

## NEUROLOGICAL DISEASES

## PSYCHIATRIC DISEASES

# PREVENTIVE
# MEDICINE

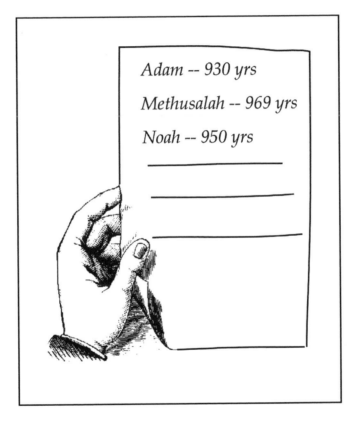

Adam -- 930 yrs

Methusalah -- 969 yrs

Noah -- 950 yrs

The first Medicare bankruptcy

# 1.1.) TYPES OF PREVENTION

| | |
|---|---|
| **primary prevention** | **= before disease is present**<br><br>○ vaccinations<br>○ prevention of nutritional deficiencies<br>○ prevention of specific injuries |
| **secondary prevention** | **= during latent disease**<br><br>○ early detection of disease<br>○ screening |
| **tertiary prevention** | **= during symptomatic disease**<br><br>○ limitation of physical and social consequences of disease<br>○ rehabilitation |

# 1.2.) CANCER SCREENING

## A) Screening Tests that are Recommended:

| | |
|---|---|
| **breast cancer** | **> 40 years:** annual clinical exam<br>**> 50 years:** mammography every 1~2 years |
| **cervix cancer** | • Pap smears every 1~3 years<br>• for all women who are or have been sexually active |
| **prostate cancer** | **> 40 years:** digital rectal exam<br>**> 50 years:** annual PSA (somewhat controversial) |
| **colon cancer** | • fecal occult blood if > 50 years or family history<br>• **colonoscopy if family history of polyposis** |
| **testicular cancer** | • if history of **cryptorchidism or testicular atrophy** |

## B) Screening Tests that are NOT Recommended:

| | |
|---|---|
| **ovarian cancer** | • routine screening **not recommended** |
| **endometrial cancer** | • routine screening **not recommended**<br>• watch for abnormal uterine bleeding in elderly women |
| **lung cancer** | • routine screening **not recommended** |

# 1.3.) <u>PREGNANCY SCREENING</u>

| | |
|---|---|
| **hypertension** | • monitor throughout pregnancy (weight gain, edema, blood pressure) |
| **Rh incompatibility** | • determine at first prenatal visit |
| **rubella titer** | • determine at first prenatal visit |
| **STDS** | <u>**screen at first prenatal visit:**</u><br>○ gonorrhea<br>○ syphilis<br>○ chlamydia<br>○ HBsAg<br>○ offer HIV |
| **bacteriuria** | • urine culture at first prenatal visit<br>• treat bacteriuria, even if asymptomatic |
| **triple screen** [1] | • at 16~20 weeks |
| **oral glucose tolerance** | • at 24~28 weeks |
| **RhoGAM vaccine** | • at 28~32 weeks if mother Rh-negative |
| **amniocentesis** | • consider for women > 35 |

[1] $\alpha$-FP , hCG , estriol

# 1.4.) <u>IMMUNIZATIONS FOR ADULTS</u>

| | |
|---|---|
| **Td booster** | • every 10 years |
| **measles** | • if born before 1957: assume "natural" immunity<br>• if born after 1957: recommend 2 doses<br><br>• protective if given within 72 h of exposure<br>• pregnant or immune compromised: give IgG |
| **Pneumovax**<br>(give once) | • elderly > 65 years<br>• chronic ill persons: COPD, HIV, CHF, DM etc.<br>• prior to splenectomy |
| **influenza**<br>(every autumn) | **now recommended to everyone, especially:**<br>• chronic ill persons: COPD, HIV, CHF, DM etc.<br>• health care professionals<br><br>• nasal = live vaccine |

 *No live vaccines for HIV positive infants or adults <u>except MMR</u>!*

*To prevent cervical cancer: **Human papilloma virus vaccine**
(HPV) recommended before onset of sexual activity: 3 doses.
(Minimum age: 9 years)*

# 1.5.) <u>IMMUNIZATIONS FOR INFANTS</u>

|  | birth | 2m | 4m | 6m | 15m | 4-6y |
|---|---|---|---|---|---|---|
| **hepatitis B** | ✓ | ✓ |  | ✓ |  |  |
| **rotavirus** |  | ✓ | ✓ | ✓ |  |  |
| **DTaP** |  | ✓ | ✓ | ✓ | ✓ | ✓ |
| **haemophilus influenzae pneumococcal** |  | ✓ | ✓ | ✓ | ✓ |  |
| **iPV (Salk)** |  | ✓ | ✓ |  | ✓ | ✓ |
| **MMR + Varicella** |  |  |  |  | ✓ | ✓ |

 *If mother positive for HBsAg also give immunoglobulins to newborn!*

*Seasonal influenza vaccine now recommended for all:*
*Minimum age 6 month (or 2 years for live, attenuated vaccine).*

**DTaP** = **D**iphtheria, **T**etanus, **a**cellular **P**ertussis

---

**Oral Polio (Sabin):**
- live-attenuated
- lifelong immunity
- local gut and systemic immunity
- may cause paralytic disease
- **discontinued in US and UK**

**Injectable Polio (Salk):**
- inactivated
- requires booster every 4~5 years
- minimal gut immunity
- no risk of paralytic disease

# 1.6.) <u>TETANUS PROPHYLAXIS</u>

## <u>MANAGEMENT OF TETANUS-PRONE WOUNDS</u>:

| Immunization History | Tetanus Toxoid | Anti-Tetanus Immune Globulin |
|---|---|---|
| **<u>3 prior doses</u>** | | |
| • clean minor wound | yes if > 10 years | no |
| • other wound | yes if > 5 years | no |
| **<u>Immunization unknown or less than 3 doses</u>** | | |
| • clean minor wound | yes | no |
| • other wound | yes | yes |

# 1.7.) ETHICS

---

✓ **Competent patients** may refuse medical treatment, even if death will result.
✓ **Pregnant woman** may refuse, even if death of fetus will result

✓ **Involuntary treatment** requires   a) patient is mentally ill
                                   PLUS
                           b) danger to self or others

✓ **Confidentiality:** May be breached if significant risk to others exists:
                         (HIV positive prostitute, patient threatens to kill, child abuse)

---

✓ **Living will:** Directions for future care (when unable to make decisions)
✓ **Durable power of attorney:** designate a legal representative to make decisions

---

✓ **Minors:** Parents must give consent
  **No consent needed if:**    - emergency
                             - pregnancy
                             - treatment of sexually transmitted diseases

✓ Some States require parental consent for abortion, others do not.

✓ Self-supporting minors are considered adults → parental consent is not required.

---

✓ You are required to report any suspicion of child abuse.
✓ You must report: HIV, syphilis, gonorrhea.

✓ Consent is required for HIV testing.

---

 *Hospital physicians cannot refuse lifesaving treatment, even if patients have no insurance or cannot pay.*

# DIAGNOSIS

## STEP by STEP

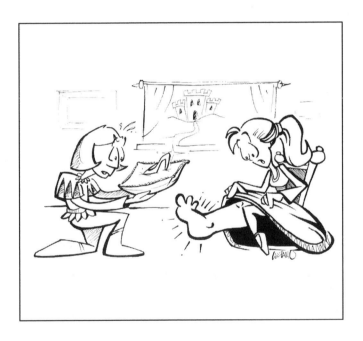

Cinderella's untimely episode of pedal edema

# 2.1.) <u>ACUTE ABDOMEN</u>

---

**1. If unstable:**

Get surgical consultation → laparotomy [1]
- perforation
- hemorrhage
- bowel obstruction
- bowel infarction

---

↓

---

**2. If stable:**

You must rule out:
- myocardial infarction
- lower lobe pneumonia
- pancreatitis
- pyelonephritis

---

↓

---

**3. If none of the above, you should consider:**
- hepatitis
- peritonitis
- diabetic ketoacidosis
- Addisonian crisis
- acute intermittent porphyria

---

[1] *increasingly replaced by laparoscopy, both diagnostic and therapeutic:*
- *cholecystectomy*
- *appendectomy*
- *adhesive obstructions*

 *Gun shot wounds → send to OR immediately!*

## 2.2.) <u>ABDOMINAL PAIN - UPPER</u>

| **1. Get ECG and chest X-ray** |
| --- |
| • myocardial infarction<br>• pericarditis<br>• pleuritis<br>• lower lobe pneumonia |

↓

| **2. Get blood chemistry** |
| --- |
| • CBC, hematocrit → serious infections, bleeding<br>• amylase, lipase → acute pancreatitis<br>• transaminases → viral or hepatocellular disease |

↓

| **3. Get upright abdominal film** |
| --- |
| • free air → perforation<br>• opacities → gall stones<br>• dilated bowel → obstruction or infarction |

↓

| **4. Consider ultrasound** |
| --- |
| • acute cholecystitis<br>• hepatic abscess<br>• subphrenic abscess |

↓

| **5. Consider upper GI endoscopy / ERCP** |
| --- |
| • gastroesophageal reflux disease<br>• peptic ulcer<br>• biliary disease |

# 2.3.) ABDOMINAL PAIN - PERIUMBILICAL

**1. Get ECG, chest X-ray and CBC**
- See 2.2. above

**2. Get abdominal flat plate or ultrasound**

**If evidence of intestinal obstruction, search for:**
- strangulation
- adhesions
- tumors
- regional enteritis

**Otherwise consider:**
- bowel infarction
- aortic aneurysm

**3. Abdominal imaging studies [1]**
- appendicitis
- diverticulitis

**4. If none of the above, you should consider:**
- Meckel's diverticulitis
- acute intermittent porphyria
- lead intoxication

[1] *CT is preferred. Barium enema is risky in case of perforated bowels.*

***Irritable bowel syndrome*** *is the most common cause of chronic abdominal pain: - at least during 12 weeks for past 12 months*
*- change in school frequency or appearance*
*- relieved after defecation*

# 2.4.) <u>ABDOMINAL PAIN - LOWER</u>

**1. Perform pelvic and rectal exam**
- ovarian cysts or tumors
- salpingitis
- ectopic pregnancy
- rectal carcinoma

↓

**2. Abdominal imaging studies (see 2.3. above)**
- appendicitis, diverticulitis
- inflammatory bowel disease

↓

**3. Non-contrast CT or IVP**
- ureteral stone or tumor

↓

**4. Consider bladder catheterization**
- if distended → obstruction

↓

**5. Consider sigmoidoscopy**
- sigmoid carcinoma
- inflammatory bowel disease
- diverticulitis

↓

**6. If none of the above:**
- irritable bowel syndrome ?

*In females of reproductive age with acute abdominal pain get a pregnancy test. If positive, verify intrauterine location with ultrasound to exclude ectopic pregnancy.*

# 2.5.) ACIDOSIS
pH < 7.35

| | |
|---|---|
| **respiratory acidosis**<br>($PCO_2$ >40 mmHg, $HCO_3$ >24 mM/L) | • hypoventilation<br>• airway obstruction<br>• decreased gas exchange |
| **metabolic acidosis**<br>($PCO_2$ <40 mmHg, $HCO_3$ <24 mM/L)<br>**anion gap > 12 mM/L** | **drug history**<br>➢ salicylate intoxication<br>➢ methanol ingestion<br>➢ ethylene glycol<br><br>**ketones present**<br>• glucose > 200 mg/dL<br>→ diabetic ketoacidosis<br>• glucose < 200 mg/dL<br>→ starvation, diet<br><br>**ketones absent**<br>• renal failure<br>• lactic acidosis |
| **metabolic acidosis**<br>($PCO_2$ <40 mmHg, $HCO_3$ <24 mM/L)<br>**anion gap < 12 mM/L**<br><br>= "hyperchloremic metabolic acidosis" | **urine pH > 5.5**<br>**renal loss of bicarbonate**<br>• carbonic anhydrase inhibitors<br>• renal tubular acidosis<br>• hypoaldosteronism<br><br>**urine pH < 5.5**<br>**GI loss of bicarbonate**<br>• diarrhea<br>• ileostomy |

# 2.6.) <u>AGITATION</u>

| | |
|---|---|
| **outburst of rage and violence** | could be another episode in a lifelong sequence of sociopathic behavior… |
| **rage and violence a/w seizure activity** | • temporal lobe seizures<br>• amygdala seizures [1] |
| **extreme freight, agitation** | **delirium**<br>• clouded consciousness<br>• psychomotor over-activity<br>• hallucinations<br><br>**anxiety disorder**<br>• acute panic attack<br><br>**schizophrenia**<br>• delusions |
| **depression, anxiety, bizarre ideation** | **developing over months or years:**<br>• schizophrenia<br>• manic-depressive disorder |

[1] *may be triggered by small amounts of alcohol*

# 2.7.) <u>AIDS</u>
## Acquired Immunodeficiency Syndrome

<u>Definition</u>

HIV positive on ELISA and confirmed by Western blot
plus • CD4 < 200 cells/mm$^3$
      • or CD4 < 14%
      • or opportunistic disease

<u>Acute Retroviral Syndrome</u> :   - fever
                                - lymphadenopathy
                                - pharyngitis
                                - rash
                                - myalgia
                                - thrombocytopenia
                                - leukopenia

<u>CD4 count</u> :   - check every 6 months   if CD4 > 300
                    - check every 3 months   if CD4 < 300
                    - start PCP prophylaxis   if CD4 < 200

| | |
|---|---|
| **ELISA** | • detects antibodies against HIV<br>• seroconversion: 4~8 weeks after transmission<br>• sensitivity and specificity are >99%<br>• if positive needs to be confirmed by Western blot |
| **rapid antibody test** | • saliva or urine → gives result in 10 minutes<br>• if positive needs to be confirmed by ELISA |
| **viral load** | • measures amount virus RNA in blood<br>• can be used prior to seroconversion<br>• used to monitor therapy |

# 2.8.) ALKALINE PHOSPHATASE

> 105 U/L

| | |
|---|---|
| **high 5' nucleotidase**<br>**high γGT** | • **biliary disease**<br>• **liver disease**<br>  - metastases<br>  - hepatocellular carcinoma |
| **high serum calcium**<br>**low serum phosphate** | • osteomalacia |
| **X-ray skull** | • Paget's disease |
| **technetium bone scan** | • bone tumors<br>• metastatic disease |
| **other** | • pregnancy |

γGT is elevated in 97% of patients with liver metastases.

γGT is the most sensitive marker of liver damage caused by alcohol.

Alkaline phosphatase isoenzymes (electrophoresis) are more difficult and expensive than the indirect methods to distinguish liver disease from bone disease.

# 2.9.) ALKALOSIS

pH > 7.45

| | |
|---|---|
| **respiratory alkalosis**<br>($PCO_2$ <35 mmHg, $HCO_3$ <25 mM/L) | **hypoxia**<br>• altitude sickness<br><br>**central stimulation**<br>• anxiety → hyperventilation<br>• salicylate intoxication<br>• encephalitis |
| **metabolic alkalosis**<br>($PCO_2$ >40 mmHg, $HCO_3$ >28 mM/L)<br>**urine Cl < 10 mM/L** | **GI loss of acid**<br>• vomiting<br>• nasogastric suction |
| **metabolic alkalosis**<br>($PCO_2$ >40 mmHg, $HCO_3$ >28 mM/L)<br>**urine Cl > 15 mM/L** | **high blood pressure:**<br>• hyperaldosteronism<br>• Cushing's syndrome<br>• renal artery stenosis<br><br>**normal blood pressure:**<br>• Bartter's syndrome<br>• severe $K^+$ deficit<br><br>• diuretics |

 *Hypovolemia prevents renal bicarbonate formation.*

---

**SALICYLATE INTOXICATION:**

**Early:** metabolic acidosis + respiratory alkalosis
**Late:** metabolic acidosis + respiratory acidosis

---

# 2.10.) ALOPECIA

## 1. If scarring is present → do biopsy first!

**Infections:**
- syphilis

**Systemic diseases:**
- discoid lupus
- scleroderma / morphea
- amyloidosis
- sarcoidosis
- (many more)

**Neoplasms:**
- skin cancer
- metastatic cancer
- lymphoma

## 2. If no scarring → screen for these:

| | |
|---|---|
| **thyroid function tests:** | hypothyroidism, hyperthyroidism |
| **VDRL:** | syphilis |
| **ferritin < 10 ng/mL:** | iron deficiency |
| **ANA:** | SLE |

## 3. Also consider:
- malnutrition
- trichotillomania
- drugs

# 2.11.) ALTERED MENTAL STATE

---

**1. Is there a history of trauma? → get CT or MRI**

CT scan abnormal:
- subdural / epidural hematoma
- intracranial bleed

CT scan normal:
- concussion

---

**2. Initial workup:**

| | | |
|---|---|---|
| body temperature | → | hypo- / hyperthermia, sepsis |
| ECG | → | arrhythmias |
| ABG | → | hypoxia, hypercapnia, CO |
| electrolytes | → | hypo- / hypernatremia |
| metabolites | → | hyperglycemia |
| | | hypoglycemia |
| | | uremia |
| | | liver failure |
| | | thyroid storm |

---

**3. If negative, consider:**

| | | |
|---|---|---|
| toxic screen | → | drugs, toxins |
| EEG | → | petit mal seizure, postictal state |
| lumbar puncture | → | meningitis, encephalitis |
| | | subarachnoid bleed |
| CT or MRI | → | intracranial bleed |

Get psychiatric evaluation!

# 2.12.) SECONDARY AMENORRHEA
normal prolactin

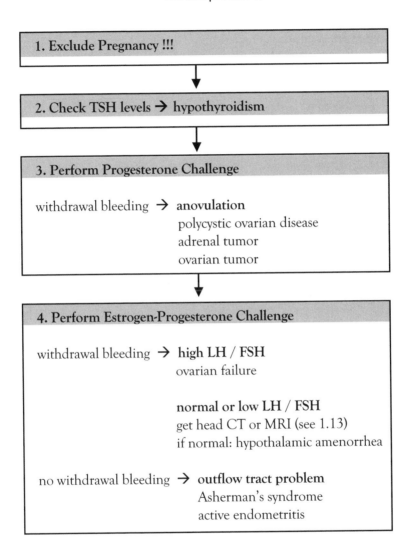

1. **Exclude Pregnancy !!!**

2. **Check TSH levels → hypothyroidism**

3. **Perform Progesterone Challenge**

   withdrawal bleeding → **anovulation**
                   polycystic ovarian disease
                   adrenal tumor
                   ovarian tumor

4. **Perform Estrogen-Progesterone Challenge**

   withdrawal bleeding → **high LH / FSH**
                   ovarian failure

                   **normal or low LH / FSH**
                   get head CT or MRI (see 1.13)
                   if normal: hypothalamic amenorrhea

   no withdrawal bleeding → **outflow tract problem**
                   Asherman's syndrome
                   active endometritis

*Any women with primary ovarian failure or ovarian failure before age 35 ("premature menopause") should be karyotyped.*

# 2.13.) <u>SECONDARY AMENORRHEA</u>
prolactin > 20 ng/mL

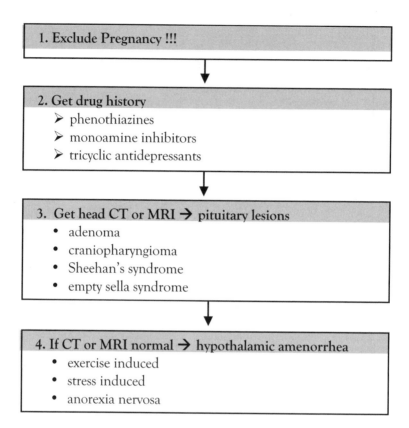

**1. Exclude Pregnancy !!!**

**2. Get drug history**
  ➤ phenothiazines
  ➤ monoamine inhibitors
  ➤ tricyclic antidepressants

**3. Get head CT or MRI → pituitary lesions**
  • adenoma
  • craniopharyngioma
  • Sheehan's syndrome
  • empty sella syndrome

**4. If CT or MRI normal → hypothalamic amenorrhea**
  • exercise induced
  • stress induced
  • anorexia nervosa

*Hypothalamic amenorrhea* is a diagnosis of exclusion. It is the most common cause of secondary amenorrhea in non-pregnant women. Prolactin levels may be normal or elevated.

# 2.14.) <u>AMNESIA</u>

## A) <u>SUDDEN ONSET</u>:

| complete recovery | <ul><li>post-concussion</li><li>TIA to hippocampal areas [1]</li><li>temporal lobe seizures</li></ul> |
|---|---|
| incomplete recovery | <ul><li>hippocampal infarction</li><li>thalamic infarction</li><li>subarachnoid hemorrhage</li><li>prolonged hypoxia</li></ul> |

## B) <u>SLOW ONSET</u>:

| incomplete recovery | <ul><li>Wernicke-Korsakoff syndrome [2]</li><li>encephalitis</li></ul> |
|---|---|
| no recovery | <ul><li>Alzheimer's disease</li><li>diencephalic tumors</li></ul> |

[1] *Patient may wonder "where am I, what's happening?"*
[2] *Memory gaps are filled in with fantastic stories (confabulation).*

# 2.15.) <u>MICROCYTIC ANEMIA</u>

MCV < 82 fL

| | | |
|---|---|---|
| **TIBC** - high<br>ferritin - low<br>iron - low | **iron deficiency**<br>• infants: decreased dietary intake<br>• elderly: occult bleed (especially GI)<br>• other: malabsorption |
| TIBC - low<br>**ferritin - high**<br>iron - low | • anemia of chronic disease [1] |
| TIBC - normal<br>**ferritin - high**<br>**iron - high** | **blocked heme synthesis**<br>• lead poisoning<br>• sideroblastic anemia |
| **electrophoresis** | • sickle cell anemia<br>• thalassemia |

[1] *can be microcytic or normocytic*

# 2.16.) NORMOCYTIC ANEMIA

MCV 82~98 fL

| | |
|---|---|
| **reticulocytes > 1.5%** | • blood loss<br>• hemolytic anemia |
| **MCHC > 36 g/dL** | • hereditary spherocytosis |
| **bone marrow biopsy** | **hypoplasia**<br>• aplastic anemia<br><br>**myelophthisis** [1]<br>• myeloma<br>• lymphoma<br>• leukemia<br>• granulomatous disease<br>• lipid storage disease<br><br>**erythroid hyperplasia**<br>• early iron deficiency |
| **other** | • chronic liver disease<br>• chronic renal disease |

[1] *myelophthisis = infiltration and replacement of bone marrow*

# 2.17.) <u>MACROCYTIC ANEMIA</u>
## MCV > 98 fL

| | |
|---|---|
| **Vit. B12 < 160 pg/mL** | **absolute B12 deficiency**<br>• pernicious anemia<br>• malabsorption<br>• ileal resection |
| **folate < 2 ng/mL** | **absolute folate deficiency**<br>• ethanol<br>• dietary |
| **bone marrow biopsy** | **normoblastic**<br>• hemolysis<br>• chronic liver disease<br><br>**megaloblastic**<br>• relative B12 deficiency<br>• relative folate deficiency<br><br>**myelodysplasia**<br>• refractory anemia<br>• CMML |

# 2.18.) HEMOLYTIC ANEMIA

| direct Coombs' test positive | **indirect Coombs' test positive:** <br> • hemolytic disease of newborn <br> • transfusion reaction <br><br> **indirect Coombs' test negative:** <br> • warm antibodies <br> • cold antibodies |
|---|---|
| **membrane abnormalities** | • spherocytosis <br> • elliptocytosis |
| **metabolic abnormalities** | • glucose-6-PD deficiency |
| **hemoglobin abnormalities** | • sickle cell anemia <br> • thalassemia |
| **mechanical trauma** | • march hemoglobinuria <br> • artificial heart valves <br> • DIC |
| **other** | • burns <br> • chemicals <br> • hypersplenism |

| WARM ANTIBODIES | COLD ANTIBODIES |
|---|---|
| • drugs <br> • infections <br> • collagen vascular diseases <br><br> • multiple myeloma <br> • lymphoma | • mononucleosis <br> • mycoplasma infection <br><br> • multiple myeloma <br> • lymphoma <br><br> • paroxysmal cold hemoglobinuria |

# 2.19.) <u>APLASTIC ANEMIA</u>

| | |
|---|---|
| **drugs: dose related**<br>(predictable) | ➢ chloramphenicol<br>➢ benzene<br>➢ chemotherapy |
| **drugs: not dose related**<br>(unpredictable) | ➢ chloramphenicol<br>➢ phenylbutazone<br>➢ sulfa drugs<br>➢ amantadine<br>➢ ACE inhibitors |
| **hereditary** | • Fanconi's anemia |
| **other** | • infections<br>• radiation |

# 2.20.) ANXIETY

| | |
|---|---|
| **drugs** | ➤ drug abuse<br>➤ medications |
| **medical conditions** | • cardiac arrhythmias<br>• hyperthyroidism<br>• pheochromocytoma |
| **objects, situations** | • specific phobia<br>• social phobia<br>• separation anxiety |
| **severe traumatic event** | **duration < 1 month:**<br>• acute stress disorder<br><br>**duration > 1 month:**<br>• post-traumatic stress disorder |
| **obsessions** | • obsessive-compulsive disorder |
| **recurrent panic attacks**<br>+<br>constant worry about attacks<br>+<br>behavioral changes to avoid<br>these attacks | • agoraphobia |

# 2.21.) <u>ARTHRALGIA</u>

## A) <u>INVOLVING SEVERAL JOINTS</u>:

> **1. If spine is <u>not</u> involved, you should consider:**
> - rheumatoid arthritis
> - psoriatic arthritis
> - SLE
>
> **2. If spine is involved, you should consider:**
> - ankylosing spondylitis
> - Reiter's syndrome

## B) <u>INVOLVING ONE JOINT</u>

### → PERFORM ARTHROCENTESIS:

> **1. If non-inflammatory**
> - bloody effusion → trauma or coagulopathy
> - non-bloody effusion → osteoarthritis

> **2. If inflammatory (synovial WBC usually > 5,000/mm³)**
> - look for crystals:
>   - positive birefringence → pseudogout
>   - negative birefringence → gout

> **3. If purulent (synovial WBC usually > 50,000/mm³)**
> **Get Gram stain or culture of synovial fluid:**
> - infectious arthritis
>   (common causes: syphilis or Lyme disease)

# 2.22.) ASCITES

## A) TRANSUDATE (SAAG > 1.1 g/dL):

**1. Check for signs of portal hypertension**
- liver cirrhosis
- congestive heart failure
- IVC obstruction

**2. Check albumin levels**
- nephrotic syndrome
- malnutrition

**3. Evidence of abdominal neoplasms? (Meig's syndrome)**
- ovarian fibroma
- ovarian cystadenoma
- struma ovarii

## B) EXUDATE (SAAG < 1.1 g/dL):

**1. Check PMN count, if >250:**
- peritonitis
  (bacterial, tuberculosis, or fungal)

**2. Check cytology**
- hepatoma, mesothelioma
- ovarian carcinoma
- metastatic carcinoma

**3. Check amylase levels**
- pancreatitis

*SAAG = (serum albumin) minus (ascites albumin)*

31

# 2.23.) <u>BLEEDING</u>

| | |
|---|---|
| **platelets < 100,000/mm$^3$** | • thrombocytopenia |
| **PT prolonged** | • Factor VII deficiency<br>• vitamin K deficiency<br>• liver disease |
| **PTT prolonged** | • Von Willebrand's disease<br>• Factor VIII (hemophilia A)<br>• Factor IX (hemophilia B)<br>• circulating anticoagulants |
| **both PT and PTT prolonged** | ➢ heparin<br>• vitamin K deficiency<br>• liver failure<br>• DIC<br>• dysfibrinogenemia<br>• circulating anticoagulants |
| **bleeding time prolonged > 10 min** | • platelet dysfunction<br>• myeloproliferative disorders<br>• uremia |

---

**MIXING STUDY:**
Repeat PT, PTT with equal mixture of patient's and normal plasma:

| | |
|---|---|
| **If times correct** | → factor deficiency |
| **If times do not correct** | → factor inhibition |

# 2.24.) <u>BRADYCARDIA</u>

< 60 beats/min

---

**1. Check drug history for causes of bradycardia**
- ➤ digitalis
- ➤ beta-blockers
- ➤ calcium channel blockers

---

**2. Obtain an ECG**

- **1st degree AV block**
  = PR > 0.2 sec.
- **2nd degree AV block, Mobitz I**
  = progressive prolongation of PR
- **2nd degree AV block, Mobitz II**
  = irregular, unexpected AV block
- **3rd degree AV block**
  = complete block

---

**3. Consider Holter monitoring**
- sick sinus syndrome

---

**4. His bundle ECG to determine need for pacemaker is recommended for patients with:**
- symptomatic bundle branch block
- 2:1 AV conduction block
- asymptomatic 3rd degree AV block

---

*Trained athletes may have <50 beats/min due to increased vagus nerve tone (=nerve firing rate).*

# 2.25.) BREAST NODULE

**1. If you have a low index of suspicion, observe for:**
- physiologic nodularity
- cyclic tenderness

**2. If a cyst is likely:**
- aspiration of fluid will be diagnostic

**3. If there is a palpable lump:**
→ perform fine needle aspiration (FNA)
(sensitive and specific)

**4. Breast biopsy is indicated if:**
- suspicious mass persists through cycle and and FNA is equivocal.
- residual component left after attempted cyst aspiration.
- suspicious mass plus spontaneous serosanguineous discharge.
- suspicious mammogram without prominent palpable mass.

*Recommend monthly breast self-examination for all women above 20 years of age.*

## BREAST SELF-EXAM:

---

### 1.

- ✓ Stand in front of a mirror and look at each breast to see if there is a lump, a depression, a difference in skin texture or any other change.
- ✓ Be especially alert for any changes in the nipples' appearance.
- ✓ Raise both arms and check for any swelling or dimpling in the skin of your breasts.

---

### 2.

- ✓ Lie down with a pillow under your right shoulder and put your right arm behind your head.
- ✓ With the pads of the fingers of your left hand, make firm circular movements over each quadrant and feel for any lumps or tenderness.
- ✓ When you reach the upper outer quadrant, continue towards your armpit.

---

### 3.

- ✓ Feel your nipple for any change in size and shape.
- ✓ Squeeze your nipple to see if there is any discharge.

# 2.26.) <u>CARDIAC MURMURS</u>

| | |
|---|---|
| **mitral stenosis** | **diastolic opening snap**<br>**diastolic rumble**<br>**loud S1**<br>**no S3 or S4**<br>• dyspnea, orthopnea<br>• atrial fibrillation |
| **mitral regurgitation** | **holosystolic murmur**<br>**may radiate to axilla**<br>**widely split S2 (early A2)**<br>• pulmonary congestion |
| **mitral valve prolapse** | **midsystolic click followed by murmur**<br>• palpitations<br>• atypical chest pain |
| **aortic stenosis** | **harsh systolic ejection murmur**<br>**may radiate to carotids**<br>• angina<br>• exertional syncope |
| **aortic regurgitation** | **diastolic decrescendo murmur**<br>• "waterhammer pulse"<br><br>**DeMusset:** head bobbing<br>**Traube:** pistol shot sounds over arteries<br>**Quincke:** pulsatile blushing of nail beds |

*Follow up with - echocardiogram*
  *- cardiac catheterization*

*Inspiration:* - *increases venous return*
            - *increases right-sided murmurs*

| | OCM | AS | MR |
|---|:---:|:---:|:---:|
| **Valsalva** (decreases venous return) | ↑ | ↓ | ↓ |
| **squatting** (increases systemic vascular resistance) (increases venous return) | ↓ | ↑ | ↑ |
| **amyl nitrate** (decreases arterial pressure) (increases cardiac output) | ↑ | ↑ | ↓ |

*OCM: obstructive cardiomyopathy,  AS: aortic stenosis,  MR: mitral regurgitation*
↑ *increases murmur,*  ↓ *decreases murmur*

| | |
|---|---|
| **physiologic split** | **P closes after A  (inspiratory split)** |
| **wide split** | **P closes after A (inspiratory >> expiratory)**<br>• pulmonary stenosis<br>• mitral regurgitation<br>• RBBB |
| **paradoxical split** | **A closes after P  (expiratory split)**<br>• aortic stenosis<br>• tricuspid regurgitation<br>• LBBB |
| **fixed split** | **split independent of respiration**<br>• ASD, VSD |

*A: aortic valve   P: pulmonary valve*

# 2.27.) CARDIOMEGALY

| Echocardiogram: | |
|---|---|
| **hypertrophy** | **asymmetrical**<br>• hypertrophic cardiomyopathy<br><br>**symmetrical**<br>• hypertension<br>• coarctation of aorta<br>• high-output state |
| **dilation** | **left ventricle**<br>• decompensation<br><br>**aortic stenosis**<br>• left ventricle and aorta<br>• aortic regurgitation<br><br>**left ventricle and left atrium**<br>• mitral regurgitation<br><br>**left atrium and pulmonary artery**<br>• mitral stenosis<br><br>**right ventricle, "pruning" of pulmonary vessels**<br>• cor pulmonale<br>• primary pulmonary hypertension<br><br>**generalized enlargement**<br>• alcohol abuse<br>• post viral |
| **pericardial** | • pericardial effusion<br>• infiltrative disease |
| **normal** | • kyphoscoliosis<br>• mediastinal mass<br>• pregnancy |

| NORMAL | DILATED |
|---|---|
| 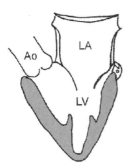 | 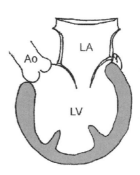 |

In the normal heart, the left intraventricular chamber is cone shaped, tapering at the apex. In dilated (congestive) cardiomyopathy, the LV chamber becomes dilated and nearly spherical in diastole.

| HYPERTROPHIC | RESTRICTIVE |
|---|---|
| 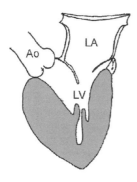 | 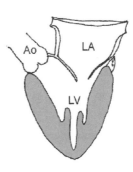 |

In hypertrophic cardiomyopathy, the LV cavity is very small in diastole, often asymmetric. In restrictive cardiomyopathy, the myocardium is very stiff and the LV cavity smaller than normal.

Modified from Chizner: *Clinical Cardiology Made Ridiculously Simple*, MedMaster, 2010

# 2.28.) CHEST PAIN

**1. Check ECG for signs of ischemia**
- cardiac enzymes elevated → myocardial infarction
- cardiac enzymes normal → angina pectoris

**2. If arterial blood gases show hypoxemia:**
**Get ventilation-perfusion scan:**
- pulmonary embolus

**Get echocardiogram:**
- aortic stenosis
- mitral valve prolapse
- cardiomyopathy
- pericarditis

**3. Get chest X-ray**
- pneumothorax
- pneumonia
- aortic aneurysm

**4. Other tests to perform if chest pain persists:**

**Treadmill, cardiac catheter, Holter monitor:**
- coronary artery disease
- arrhythmia

**Evaluate gastrointestinal tract:**
- ulcer disease
- esophageal disease
- gallbladder disease

**Also consider:**
- skeletal pain, psychogenic pain

# 2.29.) CONSTIPATION

## 1. Check drug history for causes of constipation
- anticholinergics
  (phenothiazines, antidepressants, anticonvulsants)
- narcotics
- aluminum-containing antacids
- laxative abuse (*melanosis coli*)

## 2. Search for electrolytes or metabolic causes
- hypokalemia
- hypothyroidism
- diabetes mellitus

## 3. Perform sigmoidoscopy
- anorectal fissures/strictures/abscess
- rectal carcinoma
- diverticulitis

## 4. Perform barium enema or colonoscopy
- strictures
- polyps or carcinoma

**If dilated → biopsy**
- Hirschsprung's disease
- Chagas' disease

## 5. If none of the above, consider:
- irritable bowel syndrome
- depression

# 2.30.) CHRONIC COUGH

**1. Check for signs of infection or allergy**
- bronchitis, pharyngitis
- exposure to airway irritants

**2. Chest X-ray shows a solitary lesion**
- malignancy
- fungal infection

**3. Chest X-ray shows diffuse infiltration**
Sputum culture positive:
- bacterial, fungal or parasitic infection

Sputum culture negative:
- sarcoidosis
- interstitial fibrosis
- aspiration

**4. Get pulmonary function tests**
Obstructive diseases:
- asthma
- extrinsic compression

**5. Consider bronchoscopy**
- endobronchial tumor
- foreign body

*Chest X-ray is indicated if cough is chronic or if acute without signs of upper respiratory infection.*

*ACE inhibitors can cause chronic cough.*
*→ stop medicine and observe for 4 weeks.*

# 2.31.) CYANOSIS

## A) PERIPHERAL CYANOSIS:
(Tongue is red)

| congenital | **lower extremities**<br>patent ductus arteriosus |
|---|---|
| **localized cyanosis**<br>**($O_2$ saturation normal)** | venous thrombosis<br>Raynaud's phenomenon<br>acrocyanosis |

## B) CENTRAL CYANOSIS:
(Tongue is blue)

| **$p_aO_2 > 50$ mmHg** | methemoglobin<br>(chocolate colored blood) |
|---|---|
| **$p_aO_2 < 50$ mmHg** | **$p_aO_2$ increases with 100% $O_2$**<br>lung disease<br>heart disease |
| **$p_aO_2 < 50$ mmHg** | **$p_aO_2$ does not increase with 100% $O_2$**<br>primary right → left shunt<br>Eisenmenger reaction |
| **CXR** | congestive heart failure<br>Pneumonia |
| **V/Q scan** | pulmonary embolus |

| Polycythemia | - cyanosis becomes apparent early |
|---|---|
| Anemia | - cyanosis becomes apparent late |

# 2.32.) DEMENTIA

## 1. Are focal neurological signs present?
- CNS tumors
- lacunar stroke
- multiple sclerosis

## 2. Are extrapyramidal signs present?
- Parkinson's
- Huntington's
- supranuclear palsy

## 3. Check for metabolic abnormalities
- uremia
- thyroid function tests
- hepatic encephalopathy

## 4. Do some serological tests
- syphilis
- AIDS

### 5. Perform a toxic screen
- drugs
- alcohol
- heavy metals

### 6. Consider lumbar puncture
- meningitis
- encephalitis

### 7. If none of the above, consider:
- Jacob-Creutzfeldt disease
- Alzheimer's disease
- depression

***Alzheimer's disease*** - *parietotemporal atrophy*
***Pick's disease*** - *frontotemporal atrophy*

# 2.33.) <u>DIARRHEA - ACUTE</u>

**1. If no fever or systemic signs: treat symptomatically**

**2. Check drug history for causes of diarrhea**
- laxatives
- magnesium-containing antacids
- lactulose
- antibiotics → *Cl. difficile* toxin in stool?
  (pseudomembranous colitis)

**3. Check stool for ova and parasites, or culture**
- *Cryptosporidium* (common in AIDS patients)
- *Giardia lamblia*
- Entamoeba histolytica
- worms

**4. If stool is negative for ova and parasites:**
- viral gastroenteritis

**Food poisoning:**
- *Cl. perfringens*
- *Staph. aureus*

**5. If diarrhea still persisting do sigmoidoscopy:**
- rectal carcinoma
- inflammatory bowel disease

*<u>WHEN TO ADMIT PATIENT</u>*
*- severe dehydration*
*- bloody diarrhea that gets worse*
*- severe abdominal pain (acute abdomen)*
*- high fever*
*- diarrhea in immunocompromised patient*

# 2.34.) DIARRHEA - CHRONIC

| 1. Obtain drug history and check for ova and parasites |
|---|

| 2. Perform sigmoidoscopy or barium enema |
|---|
| • carcinoma |
| • inflammatory bowel disease |
| • scleroderma |

| 3. Upper GI and small bowel series or endoscopy |
|---|
| • Crohn's disease |
| • celiac sprue |

| 4. Measure fecal fat content, if > 7 g/24h: |
|---|
| Malabsorption: |
| • celiac sprue |
| • pancreatic insufficiency |
| • blind loop syndrome |

## RESULT OF A PROLONGED FAST:

| DIARRHEA RESOLVES | DIARRHEA PERSISTS |
|---|---|
| **D-xylose absorption test:**<br>- bacterial overgrowth | **Serum or urine hormone levels:** |
| **Cholestyramine trial:**<br>- bile acid malabsorption | - carcinoid<br>- VIPoma |

# 2.35.) DIZZINESS

---

**1. Check drug history for causes of dizziness**
- tranquilizers
- antihypertensives
- antidepressants

↓

**2. Consider Holter monitoring**
- cardiac arrhythmia

↓

**3. Perform EEG**
- seizure disorder

↓

**4. If none of the above, consider:**
- posterior TIA
- hyperventilation syndrome

*Vertigo   = rotating sensation*
*Dizziness = fainting sensation*

# 2.36.) <u>DYSMENORRHEA</u>

 *Colicky, labor-like pain*

---

**1. Perform pelvic exam**
- cervical stenosis
- uterine fibroids
- presence of IUD

↓

**2. Get ultrasound**
- uterine abnormalities
- outflow obstructions

↓

**3. Consider hysterosalpingography or hysteroscopy**
- endometrial polyps

↓

**4. Consider laparoscopy**
- endometriosis
- pelvic adhesions

↓

**5. If none of the above:**
- primary dysmenorrhea
  (=absence of identifiable pelvic abnormalities)

# 2.37.) DYSPAREUNIA

## PERFORM PHYSICAL EXAM:

| | |
|---|---|
| **vaginal opening** | • residual hymen<br>• episiotomy scar<br>• Bartholin's gland abscess |
| **clitoris** | • irritations<br>• infections |
| **vagina** | • infections<br>• atrophy<br>• decreased lubrication |
| **uterus, tubes** | • endometriosis<br>• pelvic inflammatory disease<br>• ectopic pregnancy |
| **other** | • psychological |

*It is not rare for a women to overcome her dyspareunia and then find her partner becoming impotent...*

# 2.38.) <u>DYSPHAGIA</u>

---

**1. Consider esophagoscopy**
- neoplasms
- esophageal rings/strictures
- Zenker's diverticulum
- achalasia

↓

**2. Consider barium swallow (video)**
**External compression:**
- mediastinal masses
- atrial enlargement

↓

**3. Consider esophageal manometry**
**Progressive neurological disorders:**
- Parkinson's
- diabetic neuropathy
- multiple sclerosis
- syringomyelia

**Motility disorders:**
- scleroderma
- myasthenia gravis

---

 ***Painful swallowing**: pharyngitis, stomatitis*

---

**Dysphagia** = sensation of impaired act of swallowing.
**Globus** = sensation that something is stuck in the throat.

# 2.39.) DYSPNEA

| | |
|---|---|
| **CXR "pulmonary"** | • pneumonia<br>• interstitial lung disease<br>• emphysema<br>• pneumothorax |
| **CXR "cardiac"** | **echocardiogram**<br>• valvular disease<br>• myopathy |
| **$pO_2$ > 70 mmHg** | **$O_2$ saturation > 95%**<br>• CO poisoning<br>• methemoglobulinemia<br><br>**hematocrit < 35%**<br>• anemia |
| **$pO_2$ < 70 mmHg** | **V/Q scan**<br>• pulmonary embolus<br><br>**cardiac catheter**<br>• right→left shunt<br>• pulmonary hypertension |
| **pulmonary function tests (PFT)** | • airway obstruction<br>• bronchospasm<br>• restrictive disease<br>• respiratory muscle weakness |
| **exercise PFT** | • exercise induced asthma<br>• fixed cardiac output |

# 2.40.) DYSPROTEINEMIA

### monoclonal gammopathy

| | |
|---|---|
| **bone marrow abnormal**<br>( > 10% plasma cells ) | **IgM**<br>• Waldenström's macroglobulinemia [1]<br><br>**IgG, IgM,** rarely IgA, IgD, or IgE<br>• multiple myeloma [2] |
| **bone marrow normal**<br>( 1~2% plasma cells ) | **IgM (secondary macroglobulinemia)**<br>• chronic inflammation<br>• carcinoma<br>• lymphoma<br>• CLL<br><br>**urine protein electrophoresis positive**<br>• primary amyloidosis [3]<br><br>**urine protein electrophoresis negative**<br>• MGUS [4] |

[1] *lymphoma of medium-sized B cells*

[2] *malignancy of plasma cells*

[3] *diagnosis requires demonstration of amyloid on tissue biopsy*

[4] *follow monoclonal M-component with immune-electrophoresis every 6 months*

---

<u>M-component</u>:

IgG - typical myeloma
light chain (κ or λ) - more aggressive

• may precipitate in cold (cryoglobulin) → Raynaud's
• may complex with coagulation factors → coagulopathy
• appears in urine (Bence-Jones protein) in 75% of cases

# 2.41.) EDEMA

## A) GENERALIZED:

| | |
|---|---|
| **jugular vein pressure elevated** | **echocardiogram**<br>• congestive heart failure<br>• pericarditis<br>• tamponade |
| **serum albumin < 3 g/dL** | **24h urine protein > 3.5 g**<br>• nephrotic syndrome<br><br>**LFTs abnormal**<br>• hepatic failure<br><br>**prealbumin < 20 mg/dL**<br>• malnutrition |
| **thyroid function tests** | **high TSH**<br>• myxedema |

## B) REGIONAL:

| | |
|---|---|
| **upper extremity** | **jugular vein pressure elevated**<br>• superior vena cava syndrome<br><br>**Doppler or venography**<br>• venous thrombosis<br>• lymphatic obstruction |
| **lower extremity** | **Doppler or venogram**<br>• venous thrombosis<br>• lymphatic obstruction |

# 2.42.) EOSINOPHILIA

> $500/mm^3$

| allergy | <ul><li>drugs</li><li>hay fever</li><li>asthma</li></ul> |
| --- | --- |
| **skin disorders** | <ul><li>atopic dermatitis</li><li>pemphigus vulgaris</li></ul> |
| **parasites** | <ul><li>trichinosis</li><li>toxocara</li><li>echinococcus</li></ul> |
| **CXR: pulmonary infiltrate** | <ul><li>Löffler's syndrome [1]<br>(eosinophilic pneumonia)</li></ul> |

[1] *eosinophils can be found in sputum*

*Eosinophilia is more likely if tissue is invaded by parasites (e.g. trichinosis) than when parasites inhabit the visceral lumen (e.g. tapeworms).*

# 2.43.) <u>EPISTAXIS</u>

| local causes | • trauma to Little's area [1]<br><br>• nasal fracture<br>• nasal tumors<br>• septal granulomas/perforations |
|---|---|
| **systemic cause** | • hypertension<br>• coagulopathy<br>• hereditary telangiectasis<br>  (=Osler syndrome) |

[1] *most common cause of nose bleed in children*

 *It is important to identify the site of bleeding as accurately as possible in case a vessel needs to be tied later.*

## 2.44.) RED EYE

| | ACUTE GLAUCOMA | CONJUNCTIVITIS | UVEITIS | KERATITIS |
|---|---|---|---|---|
| **conjunctiva** | conjunctival and ciliary vessels injected | conjunctival vessels injected<br><br>most marked away from corneoscleral margin | ciliary vessels injected<br><br>most marked on corneoscleral margin | conjunctival vessels injected<br><br>most marked on corneoscleral margin |
| **cornea** | hazy, insensitive | clear, sensitive | clear, sensitive | opaque, diminished reflex |
| **iris** | injected | normal | swollen, adheres to lens | normal |
| **anterior chamber** | shallow | normal | may be turbid | normal |
| **pupil** | dilated, fixed | normal | small, fixed | normal |
| **intraocular pressure** | increased | normal | normal | normal |

# 2.45.) FATIGUE

## 1. Check electrolytes and CBC
- anemia
- hypokalemia
- uremia
- diabetes mellitus
- adrenal insufficiency

↓

## 2. Check for signs of infection
- viral prodrome

**Chronic infections:**
- tuberculosis
- endocarditis
- parasitic/fungal

↓

## 3. Screen for drugs and toxins
➢ heavy metals
➢ carbon monoxide
➢ solvents

↓

## 4. Perform thyroid tests
- hypothyroidism / hyperthyroidism

↓

## 5. Search for occult malignancies

↓

## 6. If none of the above, consider:
- nutritional deficiency
- depression
- severe stress
- chronic fatigue syndrome

# 2.46.) <u>FEVER OF UNKNOWN ORIGIN</u>

| | |
|---|---|
| **CXR** | • tuberculosis<br>• lymphoma |
| **blood, urine, throat cultures** | • endocarditis<br>• sepsis<br>• etc… |
| **HIV antibody test** | • AIDS |
| **liver function tests** | • hepatitis |
| **serology** | • Lyme disease<br>• salmonella<br>• typhus<br>• psittacosis |
| **RBC thick smear** | • malaria |
| **ESR elevated** | • SLE<br>• vasculitis<br>• Still's disease |
| **echocardiogram** | • endocarditis<br>• pericarditis |
| **bone scan** | • metastatic disease<br>• osteomyelitis |
| **abdominal/pelvic CT scan** | • abscess<br>• lymphoma<br>• occult malignancies |
| **viral cultures**<br>(expensive, low yield) | • Epstein-Barr virus<br>• cytomegalovirus |

# 2.47.) FOLIC ACID DEFICIENCY

## < 2 ng/mL

| | |
|---|---|
| **inadequate intake** | ○ alcoholics<br>○ infants |
| **impaired absorption** | • steatorrhea<br>• sprue<br>• jejunal resection<br>• Whipple's disease<br>• amyloidosis |
| **impaired metabolism** | **anti-folates:**<br>➤ pyrimethamine<br>➤ trimethoprim<br>➤ methotrexate |
| **increased requirements** | • pregnancy<br>• infancy<br>• hyperthyroidism<br>• malignancy |

# 2.48.) GAIT ABNORMALITIES

| | |
|---|---|
| **cerebellar** | **wide base**<br>**swaying of trunk**<br>**difficulty walking line heal to toe**<br>• multiple sclerosis<br>• medulloblastoma<br>• cerebellar degeneration (alcoholism) |
| **sensory ataxia** | **Romberg sign (patient falls when closing eyes)**<br>**patient stomps feet**<br>**patient watches feet and ground closely**<br>• damage to posterior roots/columns<br>• tabes dorsalis<br>• vit. B12 deficiency<br>• multiple sclerosis |
| **labyrinthine** | **can't focus vision when moving**<br>**must stop to read signs** |
| **Parkinson** | **involuntary acceleration**<br>**rigid, shuffling**<br>**"patient chases his center of gravity"** |
| **equine gait**<br>**(foot drop)** | **excessive hip flexion to compensate**<br>• peroneal nerve damage<br>• poliomyelitis<br>• Charcot-Marie-Tooth disease<br>• (peroneal muscle atrophy) |
| **waddling gait** | **failure to stabilize weight bearing hip**<br>• weakness of gluteal muscles<br>• muscular dystrophy |
| **drunken gait** | **reels and swamps in many directions**<br>**patient seems unconcerned** |
| **hysterical gait** | **"stiff leg"**<br>**exaggerated, dystonic posturing** |

# 2.49.) GASTROINTESTINAL BLEEDING

| | |
|---|---|
| **hematemesis** | **upper GI endoscopy**<br>• esophageal varices<br>• Mallory-Weiss tear<br>• gastric ulcer<br>• duodenal ulcer |
| **hematochezia / melena** | **upper GI endoscopy**<br>(as above)<br><br>**colonoscopy**<br>• infectious colitis<br>• inflammatory bowel disease<br>• neoplasms<br>• ischemic bowel<br><br>**angiography**<br>• neoplasms<br>• angiodysplasia (malformation) |
| **bright red blood per rectum** | **hemorrhoids**<br>• fissures<br><br>**sigmoidoscopy then colonoscopy**<br>• infectious colitis<br>• inflammatory bowel disease<br>• neoplasms<br>• diverticulitis |
| **occult blood** | **evaluate hematocrit and iron**<br><br>**colonoscopy**<br>**upper GI endoscopy** |

# 2.50.) <u>GYNECOMASTIA</u>

| | |
|---|---|
| **neonatal** | **physiologic**<br>• 70% of male neonates<br>• placental estrogens<br>• hCG stimulation of Leydig cells |
| **puberty** | **physiologic**, often one-sided<br>• constitutional sensitivity to estrogen<br><br>**pathologic**<br>• testicular feminization<br>   - androgen insensitivity |
| **adults** | **drugs**<br>➢ spironolactone<br>➢ cimetidine<br>➢ marijuana<br><br>**pathologic**<br>• bronchogenic carcinoma<br>   - ectopic hCG production<br>• liver disease<br>   - reduced estradiol metabolism<br><br>• Leydig cell tumor |
| **elderly** | **physiologic**<br>• decreased testosterone<br>   - imbalance in ratio of free testosterone<br>    to free estrogen |

# 2.51.) ACUTE HEADACHE

## A) SUDDEN ONSET:

| recent trauma | no focal signs → observe |
| --- | --- |
| | focal signs → MRI<br>• epidural hemorrhage [1] |
| no trauma | MRI<br>• subarachnoid hemorrhage |

## B) GRADUAL ONSET:

| history of trauma | MRI scan<br>• subdural hemorrhage [2] |
| --- | --- |
| fever plus nuchal rigidity<br>or<br>fever plus focal signs | lumbar puncture<br>• meningitis<br>• encephalitis |
| no fever | MRI scan<br>• tumors<br>• brain abscess<br>• intracranial bleed |

[1] *headache, confusion or focal signs appear several hours after injury*
[2] *similar to epidura, but longer latency*

# 2.52.) CHRONIC HEADACHE

| | |
|---|---|
| **unilateral, throbbing** | **aura**<br>• classic migraine [1]<br><br>**no aura**<br>• common migraine [1] |
| **unilateral, non-throbbing** | **lacrimation, rhinorrhea**<br>• cluster headache<br><br>**tender temporal artery**<br>• temporal arteritis |
| **bilateral, non-throbbing** | • tension headache |
| **other** | • hypertensive headache |

[1] *usually throbbing, typically but not always unilateral*

 *Consider temporal arteritis in all patients >50 years.*
*Early diagnosis prevents visual loss.*

# 2.53.) <u>HEARING LOSS</u>

| | |
|---|---|
| **conductive deafness** | **Weber test: lateralizes to sick ear**<br>**Rinne test:  negative (can't hear)**<br><br>• occlusion of external auditory canal<br>• cholesteatoma<br>• chronic otitis<br>• otosclerosis |
| **nerve deafness** | **Weber test: lateralizes to healthy ear**<br>**Rinne test: positive (can hear)**<br><br>• cochlear disease<br>• cochlear nerve damage |
| **central deafness** | **brainstem evoked auditory potentials (BAEP)**<br>• damage to cochlear nuclei |

*Weber test*: Place tuning fork on top of skull.
***Rinne test***: *Place tuning fork on mastoid process. When sound ceases, hold next to auditory meatus (patient should be able to hear again).*

***BAEP*** *is a very sensitive measure to detect acoustic neuromas or other tumors of cerebellopontine angle.*

# 2.54.) HEMATURIA

| | |
|---|---|
| **white cell casts** | • pyelonephritis |
| **red cell casts** | • SLE<br>• chronic glomerulonephritis |
| **urine culture** | • cystitis<br>• pyelonephritis<br>• prostatitis<br>• TB |
| **urine protein < 1 g/24h** | **CT or MRI**<br>• tumor, cyst, stones<br>• papillary necrosis<br><br>**cystoscopy**<br>• bladder cancer<br>• cystitis<br><br>**renal arteriogram**<br>• AV-malformation<br>• renal infarction<br>• tumors |
| **urine protein > 1 g/24h** | **if renal biopsy abnormal:**<br>• glomerulonephritis<br>• interstitial nephritis<br>• vasculitis<br><br>**if renal biopsy unremarkable:**<br>• benign familial hematuria<br>• runner's hematuria |

*Cystoscopy has ~90% sensitivity to detect bladder cancer.*
*Urine cytology has ~70% sensitivity to detect bladder cancer.*

# 2.55.) HEMOPTYSIS

**1. Get coagulation workup**
- coagulopathy
- thrombocytopenia
- leukemia

**2. Chest X-ray → solitary lesion**
- carcinoma
- granuloma
- bronchogenic cyst

**Chest X-ray → diffuse infiltrate**
**if culture positive:**
- bacterial, fungal, parasitic

**if culture negative:**
- pulmonary sequestration
- hemorrhagic telangiectasis

**3. Check ECG for valvular disease**
- mitral stenosis / pulmonic stenosis

**4. Consider bronchoscopy**
- bronchitis
- neoplasm
- foreign body

**5. Consider pulmonary angiogram:**
- pulmonary embolus / infarction
- AV fistula

# 2.56.) HEPATOMEGALY

**1. Get serology**
- HAV, HBV, HCV
- cytomegalovirus

↓

**2. Increased central vein pressure?**
- congestive heart failure
- constrictive pericarditis
- tricuspid regurgitation

↓

**3. Get CT or MRI scan**
- cysts (echinococcus etc.)
- hepatocellular carcinoma
- metastases

↓

**4. Consider liver biopsy**
- ➤ toxic or alcoholic hepatitis

- $\alpha$1-antitrypsin deficiency
- Wilson's disease
- Gaucher's disease
- lymphoma

↓

**5. Consider venogram:**
- Budd-Chiari syndrome
  (obstruction of hepatic veins)

# 2.57.) HIRSUTISM

**1. Check drug history for causes of hirsutism**
- ➤ anabolic steroids
- ➤ minoxidil

**2. Check testosterone → if elevated:**

**If serum cortisol elevated:**
- Cushing's syndrome

**Get pelvic ultrasound or CT:**
- adrenal tumors
- ovarian tumors

**Perform ACTH stimulation test:**
- congenital adrenal hyperplasia

**3. Check prolactin → if elevated:**
- ➤ chlorpromazine
- ➤ phenothiazine
- pituitary adenoma

**4. Get pelvic ultrasound**
- polycystic ovary disease

**5. If none of the above, consider:**
- porphyrias
- "idiopathic"

# 2.58.) HYPERCALCEMIA

$Ca^{2+} > 10$ mg/dL

| albumin > 5.2 g/dL | **ionized calcium normal:**<br>• pseudohypercalcemia |
|---|---|
| **drugs** | ➤ thiazide diuretics |
| **PTH elevated** | **primary hyperparathyroidism:**<br>• parathyroid adenoma<br>• MEN 1<br>• MEN 2<br><br>**secondary hyperparathyroidism:**<br>• renal failure<br>• malabsorption |
| **vit. D elevated** | • vit. D intoxication |
| **other** | **increased bone release:**<br>• immobilization<br>• malignancy<br><br>• milk-alkali syndrome |

# 2.59.) HYPERCAPNIA

$CO_2 > 45$ mm Hg

| | |
|---|---|
| **chest trauma** | • flail chest<br>• airway obstruction |
| **pH > 7.4** | **metabolic alkalosis with respiratory compensation** |
| **HCO$_3$ > 29 mM/L** | **chronic respiratory acidosis**<br>• COPD<br>• interstitial lung disease<br>• kyphoscoliosis<br>• poliomyelitis<br>• amyotrophic lateral sclerosis<br>• muscular dystrophy |
| **CXR** | **parenchymal lung disease**<br>• pneumonia<br>• ARDS<br>• pulmonary edema<br>• pulmonary embolus |
| **low expiratory pressure** | **neuromuscular weakness**<br>• botulism<br>• Guillain-Barré syndrome<br>• myasthenia gravis |
| **low FEV$_1$** | **obstructive disease**<br>• asthma<br>• bronchospasm |
| **other** | • drugs<br>• loss of respiratory drive (CNS) [1] |

---

[1] *Do NOT give 100% $O_2$ to patients with chronic hypoxia!*

# 2.60.) HYPERKALEMIA

$K^+ > 5.5$ mM/L

| | |
|---|---|
| **WBC** > **100,000/mm$^3$**<br>or<br>**platelets** > **1,000,000/mm$^3$** | **pseudohyperkalemia**<br>• leukocytosis<br>• thrombocytosis |
| **drugs** | ➤ digitalis<br>➤ ACE inhibitors<br>➤ K sparing diuretics |
| **urine K$^+$ > 20 mM/L** | **increased K$^+$ load**<br>• dietary<br>• GI bleeding<br>• massive blood transfusion<br><br>**transcellular shift**<br>• acidosis<br>• hyperglycemia/insulin deficiency<br><br>**CPK or uric acid elevated**<br>• rhabdomyolysis<br>• tumor lysis |
| **urine K$^+$ < 20 mM/L** | **low aldosterone**<br>• hypoaldosteronism<br><br>**high creatinine**<br>• renal failure<br><br>**defective tubular K$^+$ secretion**<br>• obstructive nephropathy<br>• amyloidosis<br>• SLE |

# 2.61.) HYPERLIPIDEMIA

| | |
|---|---|
| **triglycerides high**<br>cholesterol normal | **primary hyperlipidemia**   `type I`<br><br>**secondary**<br>• diabetes |
| **cholesterol high**<br>triglycerides normal | **primary hyperlipidemia**   `type IIa`<br><br>**secondary**<br>• renal failure<br>• liver disease<br>• porphyria |
| **cholesterol high**<br>**triglycerides high** | **other primary hyperlipidemias**<br><br>**secondary**<br>• diabetes mellitus<br>• nephrotic syndrome<br>• Cushing's syndrome |

---

### Increased risk for CHD if:

- Triglyceride > 200 mg/dL

- Cholesterol > 240 mg/dL
- LDL > 160 mg/dL
- HDL < 35 mg/dL

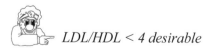 *LDL/HDL < 4 desirable*

# 2.62.) HYPERNATREMIA

$Na^+ > 145$ mM/L

---

**1. Assess volume status:**
- pulse, skin turgor, mucous membranes

---

**hypovolemia**

**urine $Na^+$ < 10 mM/L**
- diarrhea
- sweating

**urine $Na^+$ > 20 mM/L**
- osmotic diuresis
- ➢ diuretics

**volume normal**

**urine osmolarity high**
- respiratory loss
- skin loss

**urine osmolarity low**
- central diabetes insipidus
- renal diabetes insipidus

**hypervolemia**

**iatrogenic hypernatremia**
- ➢ hypertonic saline
- ➢ hypertonic $NaHCO_3$

# 2.63.) HYPERPHOSPHATEMIA

$PO_4 > 5$ mg/dL

## A) IF URINE PHOSPHATE > 1,500 mg/24h:

| | |
|---|---|
| **increased cell turnover** (CPK, LDH, uric acid elevated) | • hemolysis<br>• leukemia<br>• tumor lysis<br>• rhabdomyolysis |
| **increased load** | • transfusion of stored blood<br>• vit. D intoxication |
| **redistribution** | • acidosis<br>• hyperglycemia/insulin deficiency |

## B) IF URINE PHOSPHATE < 1,500 mg/24h:

| | |
|---|---|
| **creatinine clearance < 25 mL/min** | • renal failure |
| **Ca$^{2+}$ < 8.5 mg/dL** | **PTH low**<br>• hypoparathyroidism<br><br>**PTH normal**<br>• pseudohypoparathyroidism |
| **other** | • hyperthyroidism<br>• tumor calcinosis |

 *Decreased renal clearance is the most common cause of hyperphosphatemia.*

# 2.64.) HYPERTENSION

## A) GENERAL WORKUP:

| 1. Check drug history for causes of hypertension |
| --- |
| ➢ oral contraceptives |
| ➢ sympathomimetics |
| ➢ cocaine |
| ➢ glucocorticoids |
| ➢ mineralocorticoids |

| 2. If $K^+$ < 3.5 mM/L: |
| --- |
| Check plasma renin → if low: |
| • primary hyperaldosteronism |

## B) IF AGE OF ONSET > 30 YEARS:

| 1. Therapeutic trial → if adequate control: |
| --- |
| o most likely "essential hypertension" |

| 2. Therapeutic trial → if inadequate control: |
| --- |
| • evaluate for secondary hypertension (see section C) |

## C) IF AGE OF ONSET < 30 YEARS
### Evaluate for secondary hypertension:

---

**1. Perform dexamethasone suppression test**
- if abnormal → Cushing's syndrome

↓

**2. Check serum catecholamines**
- if elevated → pheochromocytoma
- if borderline and clonidine suppression negative → pheochromocytoma

↓

**3. Check renin → if elevated perform angiogram**
- renal artery stenosis

↓

**4. If none of the above:**
- o most likely "essential hypertension"

# 2.65.) HYPOCALCEMIA

$Ca^{2+} < 8.4$ mg/dL

| | |
|---|---|
| **albumin < 4 g/dL** | **ionized $Ca^{2+}$ normal**<br>• reduction in protein bound $Ca^{2+}$ only |
| **low PTH** | • hypoparathyroidism<br>(head and neck surgery) |
| **low phosphate**<br>**low vit. D** | **decreased $Ca^{2+}$ intake**<br>• nutritional deficiency<br>• malabsorption<br><br>**decreased vit. D production**<br>• renal disease<br>• liver disease<br>• rickets<br>• pseudohypoparathyroidism |
| **other** | ○ acute pancreatitis<br>○ hyperphosphatemia |

# 2.66.) HYPOGLYCEMIA

< 50 mg/dL

| | |
|---|---|
| **drugs** | ➤ insulin<br>➤ sulfonylureas<br>➤ beta-blockers |
| **food tolerance test** | **postprandial hypoglycemia**<br>• early diabetes mellitus<br>• dumping syndrome<br>o "idiopathic" |
| **72h fast: low glucose, high insulin** | **elevated C-peptide**<br>• insulinoma<br><br>**low C-peptide**<br>➤ insulin (factitious)<br>• insulin antibodies |
| **72h fast: high glucose, low insulin** | **insulin resistance**<br>• obesity<br>• polycystic ovary disease<br>• pregnancy |
| **other** | **artifact**<br>• leukocytosis etc. [1] |

[1] *low glucose levels in whole blood, but normal in serum.*

# 2.67.) HYPOKALEMIA

$K^+ < 3.5$ mM/L

| | |
|---|---|
| **drugs** | ➢ diuretics |
| **urine K⁺ > 20 mM/L** | **ELEVATED BLOOD PRESSURE:**<br><br>**high renin**<br>• renal artery stenosis<br>• malignant hypertension<br>• renin-secreting tumors<br><br>**low renin**<br>• hyperaldosteronism<br>• Cushing's syndrome |
| | **METABOLIC ACIDOSIS:**<br>• renal tubular acidosis |
| | **METABOLIC ALKALOSIS:**<br><br>**urine Cl⁻ < 10 mM/L**<br>• vomiting<br><br>**urine Cl⁻ > 20 mM/L**<br>• Bartter's syndrome<br>• osmotic diuresis |
| **urine K⁺ variable** | **increased cell uptake**<br>• leukemia<br>➢ insulin |
| **urine K⁺ < 20 mM/L** | **decreased intake**<br>• starvation, anorexia<br><br>**GI loss**<br>• laxatives, diarrhea |

# 2.68.) HYPONATREMIA
Na$^+$ < 135 mM/L

| | |
|---|---|
| **serum osmolality**<br>**> 295 mosm/kg** | **pseudohyponatremia**<br>• hyperglycemia<br>• hyperlipidemia |
| **edema**<br>(total body Na$^+$ increased) | **urine Na$^+$ > 20 mM/L**<br>• renal failure<br><br>**urine Na$^+$ < 10 mM/L**<br>• congestive heart failure<br>• nephrotic syndrome<br>• cirrhosis |
| **dehydration**<br>(total body Na$^+$ decreased) | **urine Na$^+$ > 20 mM/L**<br>• renal loss<br>  - diuretic excess<br>  - osmotic diuresis<br>  - ketonuria<br>• adrenal insufficiency<br><br>**urine Na$^+$ < 10 mM/L**<br>• GI loss<br>• third space loss |
| **other** | ○ psychogenic polydipsia<br><br>• SIADH [1]<br>• CNS lesions<br>• small cell carcinoma<br>• non-malignant pulmonary diseases |

[1] *severe pain, nausea and stress also stimulate ADH release*

# 2.69.) HYPOPHOSPHATEMIA

$PO_4 < 2.5$ mg/dL

| | |
|---|---|
| **intracellular/extracellular shift** | • alkalosis<br>➤ insulin |
| **urine PO$_4$ < 100 mg/24h** | **decreased intake**<br>• alcoholism<br>• malabsorption<br>• phosphate binders<br>• vit. D deficiency |
| **urine PO$_4$ > 100 mg/24h** | **hyperparathyroidism**<br><br>**tubular defects**<br>• Fanconi syndrome<br>• vit. D resistant rickets<br>➤ diuretics |

# 2.70.) HYPOTENSION

## A) ORTHOSTATIC HYPOTENSION:

| intravascular volume decreased | blood loss<br>dehydration<br>adrenal insufficiency<br><br>**shock**<br>• anaphylactic<br>• septic<br>• toxic shock syndrome<br><br>**third space loss of fluid**<br>• ascites<br>• pleural effusion<br>• edema |
|---|---|
| drugs | ➤ diuretics<br>➤ calcium channel blockers<br>➤ nitroglycerin<br>➤ phenothiazines<br>➤ tricyclic antidepressants |

## B) NON-ORTHOSTATIC HYPOTENSION:

| pale, sweating | • vasovagal hypotension |
|---|---|
| cardiovascular signs | • heart failure<br>• valvular disease<br>• pericardial tamponade<br>• arrhythmia |
| intravascular volume decreased | (see above) |

# 2.71.) URINARY INCONTINENCE

| | |
|---|---|
| **stress incontinence**<br>(coughing, strain) | **voiding cystourethrogram**<br>• urethral hypermobility (90%)<br>• damaged internal sphincter (10%) |
| **urge incontinence**<br>"uninhibited bladder" | **urinalysis / culture**<br>• bacterial cystitis<br><br>**cystoscopy**<br>• bladder tumor<br>• urethral obstruction (prostate!) |
| **overflow incontinence** | • diabetic neuropathy<br>• multiple sclerosis<br><br>**drugs**<br>➢ anticholinergics |
| **other** | • fistulae: continuous incontinence |

# 2.72.) <u>INSOMNIA</u>

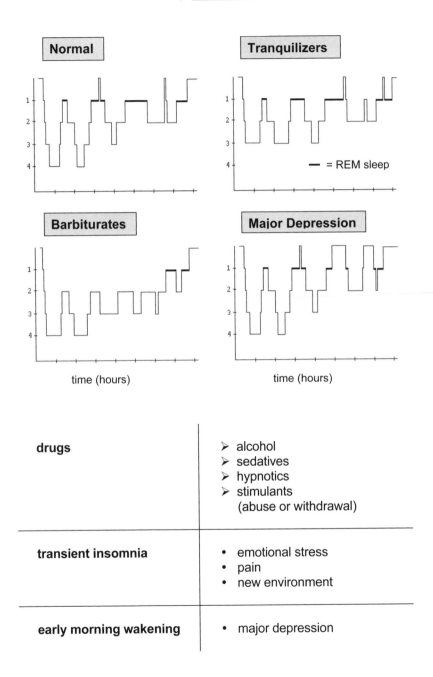

**Normal**

**Tranquilizers**

— = REM sleep

**Barbiturates**

**Major Depression**

time (hours)　　　　　time (hours)

| | |
|---|---|
| **drugs** | ➢ alcohol<br>➢ sedatives<br>➢ hypnotics<br>➢ stimulants<br>　(abuse or withdrawal) |
| **transient insomnia** | • emotional stress<br>• pain<br>• new environment |
| **early morning wakening** | • major depression |

# 2.73.) JAUNDICE

## A) UNCONJUGATED BILIRUBIN > 0.4 mg/dL

| | |
|---|---|
| **hereditary** | **transferase deficiency**<br>• Gilbert's syndrome<br>• Crigler-Najjar syndrome |
| **neonatal** | **immature transferase** |
| **drugs** | **acquired transferase deficiency**<br>➤ chloramphenicol<br>➤ pregnanediol |
| **hematocrit < 38** | • hemolytic anemia |
| **no evidence of hemolysis** | • lipid-poor hyperalimentation |

*In most hepatocellular diseases, bilirubin excretion is more impaired than bilirubin conjugation. Therefore, conjugated hyperbilirubinemia is more common.*

## B) <u>CONJUGATED BILIRUBIN > 0.4 mg/dL</u>

| | |
|---|---|
| **drugs** | ➤ oral contraceptives<br>➤ chlorpromazine<br>➤ erythromycin<br>➤ isoniazid<br>➤ halothane<br>➤ phenytoin |
| **alk. phosphatase > 300 U/L** | **ultrasound: dilated bile duct**<br>• stones<br>• sclerosing cholangitis<br>• pancreatic tumor<br><br>**CT scan / MRI**<br>• cirrhosis<br>• tumor metastasis<br>• granulomas<br><br>**other**<br>• viral hepatitis<br>• primary biliary cirrhosis |
| **ALT or AST > 300 U/L** | **viral serologies**<br>• viral hepatitis<br><br>**liver biopsy**<br>• toxic hepatitis<br>• alcoholic hepatitis<br>• infiltrative disease<br>• primary biliary cirrhosis |
| **ALT or AST < 300 U/L** | • Dubin-Johnson syndrome<br>• Rotor syndrome |

# 2.74.) LOWER BACK PAIN

**1. Get skeletal X-ray series**
- osteoarthritis
- compression fracture
- ankylosing spondylitis

**Bone diseases:**
- osteomalacia
- osteoporosis

**2. Get CT or MRI scan:**
- spinal tumors
- disc herniation
- vertebral compression fracture

**3. Abnormal physical exam (imaging normal)**
- pancreatitis
- lumbosacral strain

**4. ESR elevated (imaging normal)**
- polymyalgia rheumatica

**5. If none of the above, consider:**
- o malingering

# 2.75.) LYMPHADENOPATHY

## A) GENERALIZED:

| | |
|---|---|
| **CBC abnormal** | • lymphoma<br>• leukemia |
| **CBC variable** | • connective tissue diseases<br><br>**infections:**<br>• AIDS<br>• TB<br>• syphilis |
| **CBC normal** | • Whipple's disease<br>• sarcoidosis<br>• lipid storage disease |

## B) LOCALIZED:

| | |
|---|---|
| **head/neck** | • head/neck cancer<br>• lymphoma |
| **supraclavicular** | • lung cancer<br>• stomach cancer<br>• breast cancer |
| **axillary** | • breast cancer<br>• lung cancer |
| **inguinal** | • rectal cancer<br>• prostate cancer<br>• gynecological cancer |
| **biopsy negative** | **local inflammation:**<br>• Kawasaki's disease |

# 2.76.) LYMPHOCYTOSIS

> $4,000/mm^3$

| | |
|---|---|
| **atypical lymphocytes** | **heterophile ab test positive:**<br>• mononucleosis (EBV)<br><br>**heterophile ab test negative:**<br>• mononucleosis (CMV)<br>• hepatitis |
| **lymphadenopathy**<br>**splenomegaly** | • infections<br>• leukemia<br>• lymphoma |
| **bone marrow biopsy** | • ALL<br>• CLL<br>• hairy cell leukemia<br>• multiple myeloma<br>• non-Hodgkin's lymphoma |
| **other** | • viral infections<br><br>• pertussis<br>• tuberculosis<br>• syphilis |

 *Viral infections more commonly than bacterial cause lymphocytosis.*

# 2.77.) <u>METABOLIC SYNDROME</u>

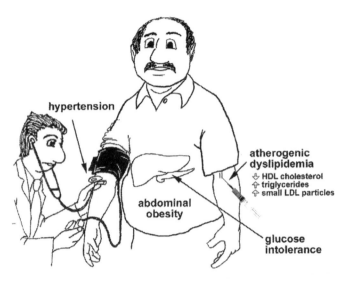

From Chizner: *Clinical Cardiology Made Ridiculously Simple*, MedMaster, 2010

---

### <u>"Metabolic Syndrome", if at least three of these are present</u>:

- Waist circumference >40 inches (men) or >35 inches (women)
- Triglycerides >150 mg/dL
- HDL cholesterol <40mg/dL (men) or <50 mg/dL (women)
- Blood pressure >130/85 mmHg
- Fasting glucose >100 mg/dL

---

*Patients with metabolic syndrome are at increased risk of coronary heart disease and diseases related to plaque buildups in artery walls and also type 2 diabetes. Probably over 50 million Americans have this!*

# 2.78.) METROMENORRHAGIA

excessive, irregular bleeding

---

**1. Pelvic exam**

**Irregular uterus:**
- myoma

**Symmetrically enlarged uterus:**
- adenomyosis
- endometrial carcinoma

---

**2. Cytologic exam:**

Not reliable for diagnosis of endometrial abnormalities. However, women in secretory phase of menstrual cycle should not shed endometrial cells.
- if abnormal → further evaluation required

---

**3. D&C = "gold standard" for diagnosis of:**
- endometrial hyperplasia vs. carcinoma

**Vabra aspirator or pipelle sampler:**
- easier and painless compared to D&C
- has become method of choice

---

*Most women have occasional menstrual cycles that are not in their usual pattern. Just observe!*

---

<u>DYSFUNCTIONAL UTERINE BLEEDING</u>:
Bleeding from proliferative endometrium as a result of anovulation in the absence of organic disease.

Recommended workup:   Pap smear
                                 Pregnancy test
                                 CBC
                                 Endometrial biopsy

# 2.79.) MONOCYTOSIS

> 750/mm$^3$

| abnormal CBC | **diagnostic bone marrow:**<br>• myeloid metaplasia<br>• leukemia<br>• multiple myeloma<br>• preleukemia<br>• lymphoma<br><br>**other:**<br>• malignant histiocytosis<br>• polycythemia vera<br>• ITP |
|---|---|
| variable CBC | **infections:**<br>• tuberculosis [1]<br>• mononucleosis<br><br>• sarcoidosis<br>• autoimmune diseases |

[1] *poor prognostic sign if monocytosis develops*

 *Infectious disease is an uncommon cause of monocytosis. Most cases are associated with hematologic disease.*

# 2.80.) MUSCLE WEAKNESS

### 1. Perform neurological exam
- Guillain-Barré syndrome
- amyotrophic lateral sclerosis
- myasthenia gravis
- porphyria

### 2. Check electrolytes and metabolic abnormalities
- hypo/hyperkalemia
- hypo/hyperthyroidism
- hypercalcemia
- Cushing's syndrome
- o familial periodic paralysis
- o familial myoglobinuria

### 3. Creatine kinase elevated?
**EMG abnormal:**
- polymyositis
- dermatomyositis

**Muscle biopsy abnormal:**
- muscular dystrophy

### 4. ESR elevated?
- polymyalgia rheumatica
- rheumatoid arthritis
- polyarteritis nodosa
- SLE

### 5. If none of the above, consider:
- depression

# 2.81.) NEUTROPENIA

< 1,500/mm$^3$

| | |
|---|---|
| **drugs** | **antibiotics**<br>➢ sulfonamides<br>➢ penicillins<br><br>➢ antihistamines<br>➢ indomethacin<br>➢ phenothiazines<br>➢ propylthiouracil<br>➢ oral hypoglycemics |
| **infections** | • sepsis<br>• viral, bacterial, parasitic |
| **splenomegaly** | • hypersplenism |
| **bone marrow biopsy** | • myelodysplastic syndromes<br>• myelophthisic syndromes<br>• acute leukemia |

# 2.82.) NEUTROPHILIA

> $10,000/mm^3$

| | |
|---|---|
| **drugs** | ➢ lithium<br>➢ digoxin |
| **reactive neutrophilia** | • infections<br>• inflammations |
| **bone marrow biopsy** | • AML<br>• CML<br>• myelofibrosis<br>• polycythemia vera |
| **other** | • post-splenectomy<br>• stress<br>○ "idiopathic" |

# 2.83.) <u>NIPPLE DISCHARGE</u>

| | |
|---|---|
| **clear or serous from multiple ducts** | ➤ oral contraceptives |
| **with pus** | • infection |
| **unilateral from single duct** | • usually intraductal papilloma<br>• rarely intraductal carcinoma |
| **prior to menstruation unilateral or bilateral** | • usually fibrocystic change |
| **milky** (increased prolactin) | **drugs**<br>➤ phenothiazines<br>➤ methyldopa<br><br>**CNS lesions**<br>• "empty sella"<br>• pituitary adenoma<br>• hypothalamic tumor |

 *Cytologic exam of nipple discharge is specific but not sensitive (i.e. negative result does not exclude carcinoma).*

 *If unilateral discharge persists → need to explore further.*

# 2.84.) <u>OLIGURIA</u>

‹ 400 mL/day

## A) $U_{Na}$ ‹ 20 mM/L, $FE_{Na}$ ‹ 1

| prerenal failure | **hypovolemia**<br>• shock<br>• blood loss<br>• third-space loss of fluid<br>• heart failure<br><br>**renal vascular resistance**<br>• malignant hypertension<br>• toxemia of pregnancy<br>• thrombosis<br><br>• hepatorenal syndrome |
| --- | --- |
| **nephritic sediment** | • acute glomerulonephritis |

 *Prerenal failure causes 80% of oliguria.*

---

### FRACTIONAL EXCRETION OF SODIUM:

Divide Na excretion by creatinine excretion:

$FE_{Na} = ( U_{Na} / P_{Na} ) / ( U_{cr} / P_{cr} )$

---

**B) $U_{Na} > 20$ mM/L, $FE_{Na} > 2$**

**1. Check urine protein, if >1 g/24h:**
**Nephritic sediment:**
- chronic glomerulonephritis

**Non-nephritic sediment:**
- vasculitis

**2. Get renal ultrasound**
**Postrenal failure:**
- stones
- neoplasms
- papillary debris
- prostatic hypertrophy
- congenital urethral obstruction

**3. Consider gallium scan, if abnormal:**
**Interstitial nephritis:**
- eosinophils → allergic
- no eosinophils → infection

**4. If none of the above, consider:**
**ATN:**
- ischemic
- toxic

# 2.85.) PANCYTOPENIA

| | |
|---|---|
| **MARROW:**<br>**hypocellular** | **marrow infiltration**<br>• lymphoma<br>• multiple myeloma<br>• TB, sarcoid, fungi<br><br>• myelofibrosis<br><br>**aplastic anemia**<br>• toxins<br>• Fanconi syndrome |
| **MARROW:**<br>**normal or hypercellular** | • myelodysplasia<br><br>• $B_{12}$ deficiency<br>• folate deficiency<br><br>• hypersplenism<br>• AIDS |
| **other** | • overwhelming infection |

# 2.86.) PARALYSIS

| | |
|---|---|
| **particular muscle group** | • **peripheral nerve damage**<br>a/w typical sensory deficits<br>severe atrophy if complete denervation |
| **monoplegia** | • **hysterical paralysis**<br>characteristic gait = "stiff leg"<br>tendon reflexes present<br>atrophy absent<br><br>• **multiple sclerosis**<br>spasticity → UMN<br>atrophy → LMN |
| **hemiplegia** | • **cortical or subcortical lesion**<br>a/w aphasia, astereognosis etc.<br><br>• **brainstem lesion**<br>a/w eye or tongue motor dysfunction<br><br>• **Brown-Séquard syndrome**<br>a/w contralateral loss of pain/temperature |
| **paraplegia**<br>(thoracolumbar cord)<br>**tetraplegia**<br>(cervical cord) | **ACUTE:**<br>spinal cord trauma<br><br>**SLOWLY PROGRESSING:**<br>**children:** muscular dystrophy<br>Friedreich's ataxia<br><br>**adults:** multiple sclerosis<br>vit. B12 deficiency<br>spinal tumors<br>syringomyelia |

# 2.87.) PLEURAL EFFUSION

| | |
|---|---|
| **cardiac exam** | • congestive heart failure |
| **thoracocentesis: transudate** | • congestive heart failure<br>• cirrhosis<br>• nephrotic syndrome<br>• hypoalbuminemia |
| **thoracocentesis: exudate** | **cytology positive**<br>• malignancy<br><br>**mononuclear cells**<br>• tuberculosis<br>• viral infection<br><br>**polymorphonuclear cells**<br>• bacterial infection<br><br>**amylase > 200 U/dL**<br>• pancreatitis<br><br>**ANA positive**<br>• SLE<br><br>**miscellaneous**<br>➢ drug reaction<br>• uremia<br>• pericardial disease |
| **thoracocentesis: blood** | • trauma<br>• malignancy<br>• pulmonary infarction |

# 2.88.) POLYCYTHEMIA

**1. Rule out pseudopolycythemia**
- dehydration

**2. Check arterial $O_2$ saturation, if < 90%:**
**High-altitude disease**
**Lung disease**
- pulmonary AV fistula
- COPD
- interstitial fibrosis
- hypoventilation

**Congenital heart disease**
- R→L shunt

**3. Check erythropoietin level, if elevated:**
**Kidney diseases**
- hydronephrosis
- polycystic kidney disease
- adenoma
- hypernephroma

**Liver tumors**

**Get hemoglobin electrophoresis:**
- abnormal hemoglobins
- methemoglobin
- carboxyhemoglobin

**4. If erythropoietin is normal:**
- polycythemia vera

# 2.89.) POLYURIA

> 3 L/day

## A) Polyuria due to solute load: urine > 300 mosm/L

**1. Search for cause**
- diabetes mellitus
- chronic renal failure
- diuretic therapy

## B) Polyuria due to water diuresis: urine < 300 mosm/L

**1. Water deprivation → if urine concentrates:**
- psychogenic polydipsia

**2. Water deprivation → if urine does not concentrate:**
- diabetes insipidus

**3. Give vasopressin**

If urine concentrates → cranial causes
- empty sella
- sella tumor
- Sheehan's syndrome

If urine does not concentrate → renal causes
- nephrotoxins
- any severe chronic renal disease

# 2.90.) PROTEINURIA

> 150 mg/24h

| urine protein < 3 g/24h | **URINE PROTEIN ELECTROPHORESIS:**<br>**light chains** [1]<br>• multiple myeloma<br><br>**albumin only**<br>• minimal change GN<br>• transient (exercise, fever)<br><br>**beta microglobulin**<br>• tubular injury |
|---|---|
| urine protein > 3 g/24h | **genetic diseases**<br>• Alport's syndrome<br>• Fabry's disease<br>• sickle cell anemia<br><br>**renal biopsy → kidney disease**<br>• glomerulonephritis<br><br>**renal biopsy → systemic disease**<br>• malignant hypertension<br>• SLE<br>• Goodpasture's syndrome<br>• Henoch-Schönlein purpura<br>• Amyloidosis |

[1] *urine dip stick false negative! (light chains do not react chemically).*

| SERUM BETA MICROGLOBULIN | URINE BETA MICROGLOBULIN |
|---|---|
| Glomerular disease<br>- diabetic nephropathy<br>- transplant rejection | Tubular injury<br>- interstitial nephritis<br>- ATN<br>- toxins |

# 2.91.) PRURITUS

### 1. Characteristic skin lesions present?
- atopic dermatitis
- allergic dermatitis

- urticaria
- folliculitis
- pemphigoid
- psoriasis
- mycosis fungoides

- lichen simplex chronicus

### 2. Check drug history
- ➢ hypersensitivity reaction
- ➢ amphetamines

### 3. Lymph nodes enlarged?
- lymphoma

### 4. Dysproteinemia?
- multiple myeloma

### 5. Abnormal liver function tests?
- obstructive biliary disease

### 6. elevated BUN / creatinine?
- uremia

# 2.92.) <u>PURPURA</u>

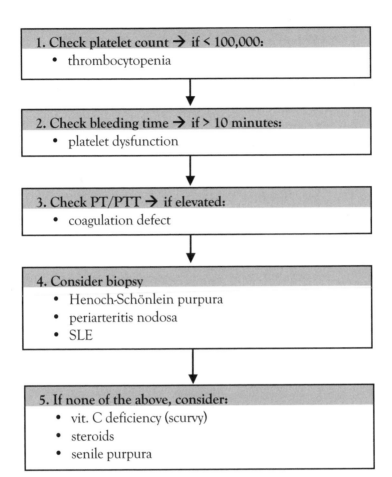

**1. Check platelet count → if < 100,000:**
- thrombocytopenia

**2. Check bleeding time → if > 10 minutes:**
- platelet dysfunction

**3. Check PT/PTT → if elevated:**
- coagulation defect

**4. Consider biopsy**
- Henoch-Schönlein purpura
- periarteritis nodosa
- SLE

**5. If none of the above, consider:**
- vit. C deficiency (scurvy)
- steroids
- senile purpura

# 2.93.) RIGHT HEART FAILURE

**1. Get Chest X-ray and ECG**
- inferior myocardial infarction

**If cor pulmonale → get pulmonary function test**
- obstructive disease (COPD)
- restrictive disease

**2. If murmurs are present → get echocardiogram**
**Valvular diseases**
- mitral stenosis
- tricuspid regurgitation
- pulmonary regurgitation
- pulmonary stenosis

**3. Consider cardiac catheterization**
**Shunt**
- atrial septal defect
- ventricular septal defect
- patent ductus arteriosus

**4. Consider V/Q scan**
- pulmonary embolus

**5. Consider Swan-Ganz catheter**
- primary pulmonary hypertension

# 2.94.) SCROTAL SWELLING

## A) PAINLESS:

| | |
|---|---|
| **hydrocele** | tense<br>fluctuant<br>**transilluminates** |
| **varicocele** | soft<br>worm-like<br>does not transilluminate<br>**collapses when patient lies down** [1] |
| **spermatocele** | vaguely circumscribed<br>does not transilluminate<br>**persists when patient lies down** |
| **tumor** | hard<br>insensitive to pressure |

[1] *if a "varicocele" does not collapse, suspect retroperitoneal neoplasm.*

## B) PAINFUL:

| | |
|---|---|
| **torsion** | young boys<br>normal urinalysis<br>→ **elevation of scrotum intensifies pain** |
| **epididymitis** | more common after puberty<br>pyuria<br>→ **elevation of scrotum reduces pain** |

# 2.95.) <u>SEIZURE</u>

**1. If there is a history of trauma → get CT or MRI**
CT scan abnormal:
- subdural hematoma
- intracranial bleed

CT scan normal:
- concussion

**2. Check blood pressure**
- hypertensive encephalopathy

**3. Search for metabolic disorders and toxins**
- hypocalcemia
- hypoglycemia
- hypoxia
- ➤ alcohol
- ➤ cocaine
- ➤ amphetamines

**4. Get EEG**
- epileptic disorder

**5. Get CT or MRI scan**
- tumors, infarction, bleeding

**6. Fever or nuchal rigidity → do lumbar puncture**
- meningitis
- encephalitis

# 2.96.) <u>SKIN RASH - ADULTS</u>

|  | RASH | OTHER SYMPTOMS |
|---|---|---|
| **drug eruptions** | - bright red<br>- intensely pruritic | 2 days ~ 2 weeks<br>after drug was given |
| **infectious mononucleosis** | - diffuse maculopapular | pharyngitis<br>lymphadenopathy<br>hepatosplenomegaly |
| **Lyme disease** | - papule, expanding to large annular<br>  lesion with central clearing | headache, myalgia<br>photophobia<br><br>arthritis weeks later |
| **typhoid fever** | - "rose spots"<br>  (small macules/papules on trunk) | abdominal pain<br>diarrhea |
| **SLE** | - erythema in sun-exposed areas<br>- "butterfly rash" | multi-organ disease |
| **2° syphilis** | - copper colored, scaly, papular,<br>- on palms and soles | primary chancre<br>still present in 10% |
| **erythema nodosum** | - large subcutaneous nodules on<br>  lower legs<br>- very tender | arthralgia |
| **Rocky Mountain spotted fever** | - maculopapular<br>- beginning on wrists and ankle<br>- spreading to trunk | fever, headache<br>myalgia |

# 2.97.) <u>SKIN RASH - CHILDREN</u>

| | RASH | OTHER SYMPTOMS |
|---|---|---|
| **measles** <br> **(rubeola)** | - discrete lesions that become confluent <br> - spreads from hairline down <br> - spares palms and soles | cough <br> conjunctivitis <br> coryza |
| **German measles** <br> **(rubella)** | - spreads from hairline down <br> - clearing while spreading | adenopathy |
| **erythema infectiosum** | - bright red <br> - "slapped cheek" appearance | mild fever |
| **exanthema subitum** | - diffuse maculopapular <br> - spares face | rash follows <br>     resolution of fever |
| **hand-foot-mouth dis.** <br> (Coxsackie virus) | - mouth: tender vesicles <br> - hands, feet: papules | fever |
| **scarlet fever** | - diffuse blanchable erythema <br> - spreads from face to trunk <br> - "sand paper" texture | fever <br> pharyngitis |

# 2.98.) SPLENOMEGALY

| CBC, ultrasound | spleen displaced by:<br>• renal mass, ovarian mass etc.<br>• metastases<br>• cysts |
|---|---|
| **congested** | • cirrhosis<br>• portal vein thrombosis/compression<br>• congestive heart failure |
| **inflammatory** | • SLE<br>• sarcoidosis |
| **infectious** | • HIV<br>• mononucleosis<br>• sepsis<br>• parasitic infections |
| **hyperplastic** | • hemolytic anemias<br>• TTP |
| **infiltrated** | • lymphoma<br>• leukemia<br>• histiocytosis X<br>• lysosomal storage diseases |
| **other** | ○ "idiopathic" |

 *A spleen palpable to med students is an enlarged spleen.*

# 2.99.) STRIDOR - CHILDREN

| congenital | choanal atresia |
|---|---|
| infections | **~2 years old:** croup |
| | **2~7 years old:** epiglottitis |
| | **any age:** diphtheria |
| | **teenager:** infectious mononucleosis |

| ACUTE EPIGLOTTITIS | ACUTE LARYNGOTRACHEOBRONCHITIS (croup) |
|---|---|
| <ul><li>rapid onset</li><li>sore throat"</li><li>child appears very ill</li><li>○ child prefers to sit upright</li><li>○ child drools saliva</li></ul> <ul><li>*H. influenzae*</li></ul> | <ul><li>1~2 days of upper respiratory infection</li><li>harsh, barking cough</li><li>chest wall recessing during inspiration</li></ul> <br> <ul><li>*parainfluenza virus, RSV, other viruses*</li></ul> |

# 2.100.) STRIDOR - ADULTS

## 1. Perform external exam
- goiter
- thyroid neoplasm

## 2. Consider laryngoscopy
- retropharyngeal abscess
- laryngitis
- diphtheria
- injury (post-endotracheal tube)

## 3. Consider bronchoscopy, biopsy
- narrowing of bronchi
- bronchial carcinoma
- mediastinal tumors
- tuberculosis/sarcoidosis

 *If stridor occurs after neck surgery, suspect damage to recurrent nerve.*

# 2.101.) SYNCOPE

---

**1. Check electrolytes, glucose, hematocrit...**
- adrenal insufficiency
- hypoglycemia
- blood loss
- dehydration

↓

**2. Check blood pressure**
- orthostatic hypotension

↓

**3. Cardiac monitoring**
- arrhythmias

↓

**4. If EEG shows seizure activity → get CT or MRI**

**If brain imaging abnormal:**
- mass lesion
- hematoma
- AV- malformation

**If brain imaging normal:**
- epilepsy

↓

**5. Attempt carotid sinus massage**
- carotid sinus syncope

↓

**6. If none of the above, consider:**
- vasovagal syncope

---

 *Distinguish from seizure, vertigo and narcolepsy!*

# 2.102.) <u>TACHYCARDIA</u>

> 100 beats/min

| | |
|---|---|
| **sinus tachycardia** | **physiologic response**<br>• (exercise, stress, hypotension etc.) |
| **atrial fibrillation** | • fever<br>• congestive heart failure<br>• thyrotoxicosis |
| **atrial flutter** | • organic heart diseases |
| **ventricular preexcitation (WPW)** | • AV bypass tracts (strands of atrial muscle around AV ring) |
| **ventricular tachycardia** | • chronic ischemia<br>• prior MI<br>• cardiomyopathy<br>➤ drug toxicity |
| **ventricular flutter/fibrillation** | • ischemic heart disease |

 ***WPW:*** *Catheter ablation of bypass tract successful in 90% of cases (recommended for both symptomatic and asymptomatic patients).*

# 2.103.) THROMBOCYTOPENIA

< 150,000 / mm$^3$

| | |
|---|---|
| **CBC** | **"artifact"**<br>• platelet clumps |
| **bone marrow:**<br>**low megakaryocytes** | **defective maturation:**<br>➢ B12 deficiency<br>➢ folate deficiency<br>➢ iron deficiency<br><br>**decreased thrombocytopoiesis:**<br>➢ drugs<br>• radiation<br>• aplastic anemia<br>• myelofibrosis<br>   - lymphoma/leukemia |
| **bone marrow:**<br>**normal or high megak's** | **myelodysplastic syndromes**<br><br>**hereditary**<br>• Wiskott-Aldrich<br><br>**PERIPHERAL DESTRUCTION:**<br>• splenomegaly<br><br>• immunological<br>   - ITP<br>   - sensitization (prior transfusions)<br><br>**PERIPHERAL CONSUMPTION:**<br>• DIC<br>• TTP<br>• hemolytic-uremic syndrome<br>• prosthetic valves |

# 2.104.) THROMBOCYTOSIS

> 400,000 / mm$^3$

| | |
|---|---|
| **> 1,000,000 platelets<br>no other abnormalities** | **"primary" thrombocythemia** |
| **bone marrow abnormal** | **myeloproliferative disorders:**<br>• polycythemia vera<br>• multiple myeloma<br>• CML<br>• myelofibrosis |
| **bone marrow reactive** | • inflammatory diseases<br>• infectious diseases<br>• acute hemorrhage<br>• carcinomas<br>• lymphomas |
| **other** | o stress<br>o exercise |

# 2.105.) <u>THYROID ENLARGEMENT</u>

| | |
|---|---|
| **goitrogens** | ➢ lithium<br>➢ iodine<br>➢ kelp |
| **low TSH**<br>**high free T4, T3** | **radioactive iodine uptake high:**<br>• Jod Basedow [1]<br>• thyroid carcinoma<br>• Graves' disease [2]<br>• Plummer's disease [3]<br><br>**radioactive iodine uptake low:**<br>• struma ovarii<br>• thyroiditis |
| **high TSH**<br>**low free T4, T3** | • endemic goiter<br>• Hashimoto's<br>➢ lithium |
| **high TSH**<br>**high free T4, T3** | • pituitary adenoma |

[1] *hyperthyroidism after administration of iodine or iodide (dietary or as contrast medium)*
[2] *diffuse toxic goiter*
[3] *multinodular toxic goiter*

## 2.106.) <u>THYROID NODULE</u>

| | |
|---|---|
| **fine needle aspiration: diagnostic** | • adenoma<br>• cyst<br><br>• papillary carcinoma<br>• follicular carcinoma<br>• medullary carcinoma |
| **fine needle aspiration: non-diagnostic** | **<u>THYROID SCAN</u>:**<br><br>**cold nodule**<br>• repeat needle aspiration or biopsy<br><br>**hot nodule**<br>• thyroid adenoma<br>• colloid adenoma |

Solitary nodules can be found in 5% of adults.
Most are benign adenomas.

**Hot nodules:**    >99% benign
**Cold nodules:**    90% benign

**Increased risk of malignancy:**    male
                                      hoarseness
                                      history of neck radiation

# 2.107.) <u>TINNITUS</u>

| | |
|---|---|
| **"crackling" noise** | • cerumen<br>• foreign body in auditory meatus |
| **"bubbling" noise** | • middle ear inflammation<br>• otosclerosis |
| **"pulsatile" noise** | • internal carotid artery thrombosis<br>• hypertension |
| **"high pitch" noise** | **cochlear damage:**<br>• exposure to excessive noise<br>• Ménière's disease [1]<br>• fracture of base of skull<br><br>**drugs:**<br>➢ aminoglycosides<br>➢ quinine<br>➢ caffeine |

[1] *tinnitus, recurrent vertigo, progressive deafness*

 *Prominent tinnitus is often the first symptom of otosclerosis!*

# 2.108.) TRANSAMINASES

normal: 0~35 U/L AST, ALT

## ELEVATED:

| | |
|---|---|
| **history of ethanol** | • ask to refrain, then repeat |
| **drugs** | ➢ oral contraceptives<br>➢ acetaminophen<br>➢ heparin<br>➢ other toxins |
| **bilirubin high**<br>**alkaline phosphatase high** | • cholestasis |
| **CPK high** | **cerebral infarction**<br><br>**acute muscle injury**<br>• IM injections<br>• severe exercise<br>• polymyositis<br><br>• acute myocardial infarction |
| **liver biopsy** | **acute hepatocellular disease**<br>• viral hepatitis<br>• infiltrative diseases<br>➢ drugs<br>➢ toxins<br>➢ alcohol |

Transaminase levels: viral hepatitis > toxic > alcoholic > tumors

# 2.109.) <u>TREMOR</u>

| | |
|---|---|
| **physiological tremor** | 10 Hz<br>(enhanced by isometric muscle contraction) |
| **enhanced physiological tremor** | • anxiety<br>• exercise<br>➢ caffeine<br>➢ alcohol withdrawal |
| **Parkinson** | • coarse, 3~5 Hz<br>• at rest<br>• forearms, hands, "pill-rolling"<br><br>**suppressed during muscle activity** [1] |
| **ataxic tremor (intention tremor)** [2] | cerebellar disease<br>**strongest during precise, exacting movements** |
| **familial tremor** | • less coarse than Parkinson's<br>• adult onset<br>• head and hands<br>➢ relieved by small amounts of alcohol [3] |

[1] *These patients can raise a full glass of water and drink its content without spilling a drop.*

[2] *Does not occur when movement is "intended" but rather when approaching intended target.*

[3] *These patients are often mistaken for alcoholics by the layperson.*

# 2.110.) <u>URTICARIA</u>

**1. If acute (< 6 weeks) consider:**
Atopic condition:
- contact urticaria
- food allergy
- drug allergy

- transfusion reactions
- serum sickness

**2. Check CBC, ANA etc.**
Autoimmune diseases:
- SLE
- connective tissue diseases

**3. Consider biopsy**
- angioedema
- vasculitis
- bullous pemphigoid

**4. If none of the above, consider:**
Physical irritation:
- heat, cold, radiation...

# 2.111.) <u>VAGINAL DISCHARGE</u>

|  | DISCHARGE | SYMPTOMS | WET SMEAR |
|---|---|---|---|
| **Candida** | thick curdy | pruritus yeast smell | hyphae |
| **Trichomonas** | thin copious | discharge | motile protozoa |
| **Gardnerella** | scant non-irritating | odor [1] | "clue-cells" [2] |

[1] *fishy odor after 10% KOH ("whiff test")*
[2] *epithelial cells with attached bacteria*

# 2.112.) VERTIGO

| | |
|---|---|
| **caloric test abnormal**<br>(labyrinthine vertigo) | **AUDIOGRAM ABNORMAL:**<br>**CT diagnostic**<br>• acoustic neuroma<br>• glomus tumor<br><br>**CT non-diagnostic**<br>• ototoxic drugs<br>• Ménière's disease<br><br>**AUDIOGRAM NORMAL:**<br>• labyrinthitis<br>• chronic otitis media |
| **spontaneous/optokinetic nystagmus**<br>(central vertigo) | **CT diagnostic:**<br>• multiple sclerosis<br>• meningioma<br>• intracranial aneurysms<br><br>**CT non-diagnostic:**<br>• vertebrobasilar<br>  insufficiency<br>• migraine |

| VERTIGO | DIZZINESS |
|---|---|
| abnormal ENG | normal ENG |
| rotating sensation<br>patient feels he is turning<br>patient feels world is turning | fainting sensation |
| nausea, visual disturbances | |

# 2.113.) VISION LOSS

| | OPHTHALMOSCOPIC FINDINGS |
|---|---|
| **retinal detachment** | **retinal bulge**<br><br>*patient describes veil over eye* |
| **macular degeneration** | **drusen** (discrete yellow deposits in macula)<br><br>*central visual loss in elderly* |
| **glaucoma**<br>ocular pressure > 20 mmHg | **enlarged central cup**<br><br>*reduced visual field* |
| **diabetic retinopathy** | • **dot-n-blot hemorrhages**<br>• **hard or cotton wool exudates**<br>• **microaneurysms**<br>• **neovascularization** |
| **hypertensive retinopathy** | • **arteriolar narrowing**<br>• **flame hemorrhages, exudates**<br>• **arteriovenous nicking**<br>• **copper and silver wiring** |
| **amaurosis fugax**<br>transient ischemic attacks | **cholesterol emboli** at arteriolar bifurcations (Hollenhorst plaques)<br><br>*transient visual loss lasting seconds* |
| **papilledema**<br>increased intracranial pressure<br>mass lesions | **blurred disc margins**<br>small cup<br>absent venous pulse<br><br>*minimal visual loss until late stage* |

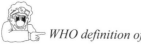 *WHO definition of blindness: vision < 1:20*

## A) Normal Retina

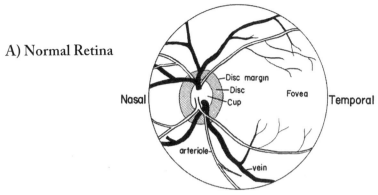

Disc margin is well-defined, disc color (shaded area) is pinkish-white. 4 groups of blood vessels spread to the 4 quadrants of eye. Veins slightly larger than arterioles.

## B) Roth Spots

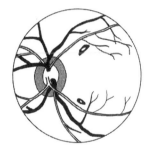

Hemorrhagic areas with whitish centers in a patient with subacute bacterial endocarditis.

## C) Retinal detachment

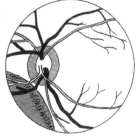

Acute onset visual loss in the left eye, like a "curtain" drawn partially over the superotemporal aspect of the visual field.

## D) Macular Degeneration

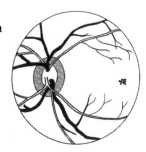

Progressive loss of visual acuity in an elderly patient. Lens is clear. Pigmental changes in foveal region.

## E) Diabetic retinopathy

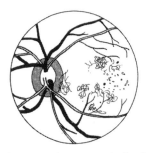

Microaneurysms, "blot" hemorrhages and neovascularisation.

## F) Hypertensive retinopathy

a.   b.   c.

**a. Normal:**  a = artery, v = vein
**b. Acute hypertension:**  exudates and hemorrhage (left), papilledema (right).
**c. Chronic hypertension:**  A-V nicking (left) and copper wiring (right).

Modified from Goldberg: *Ophthalmology Made Ridiculously Simple*, MedMaster, 2009

# 2.114.) <u>VITAMIN B12 DEFICIENCY</u>

< 160 pg/mL

---

**1. Check methylmalonic acid and homocysteine levels**
- to confirm borderline low cobalamin (100~200 pg/mL)

↓

**2. Schilling test (oral B12) is normal:**
Inadequate intake:
- breast-fed infants
- alcoholics, strict vegetarians

Increased requirements:
- cancer
- hyperthyroidism

↓

**3. Schilling test II (oral B12 plus IF) is normal:**
Lack of intrinsic factor:
- post gastrectomy
- gastric mucosal injury
- pernicious anemia

↓

**4. Schilling test III (oral B12 plus IF plus antibiotic) is normal:**
- bacterial overgrowth, "blind loop"

↓

**5. Schilling test III (oral B12 plus IF plus antibiotic) is abnormal:**
Malabsorption:
- sprue
- regional ileitis
- ileal resection

Parasites:
- fish tapeworm (*D. latum*)

Drugs:
➢ broad spectrum antibiotics

# 2.115.) <u>WEIGHT GAIN</u>

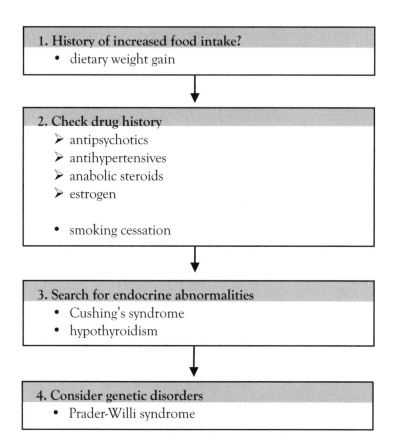

**1. History of increased food intake?**
- dietary weight gain

**2. Check drug history**
- ➤ antipsychotics
- ➤ antihypertensives
- ➤ anabolic steroids
- ➤ estrogen

- smoking cessation

**3. Search for endocrine abnormalities**
- Cushing's syndrome
- hypothyroidism

**4. Consider genetic disorders**
- Prader-Willi syndrome

# 2.116.) <u>WEIGHT LOSS</u>

**1. Psychological evaluation**
- stress, depression
- eating disorder

**2. Consider HIV test in risk patients**
- HIV

**3. Rule out endocrine disorders**
- diabetes mellitus
- hyperthyroidism
- Addison's disease

**4. Get chest X-ray**
- congestive heart failure
- COPD
- lung tumor

**4. Consider small bowel function tests**
- inflammatory bowel disease
- sprue

**5. Search for occult malignancies**
- GI tract, liver
- leukemia, lymphoma

*Hospital setting: most likely serious disease*
*Community setting: most likely stress/depression*

# THERAPY

# &

# MANAGEMENT

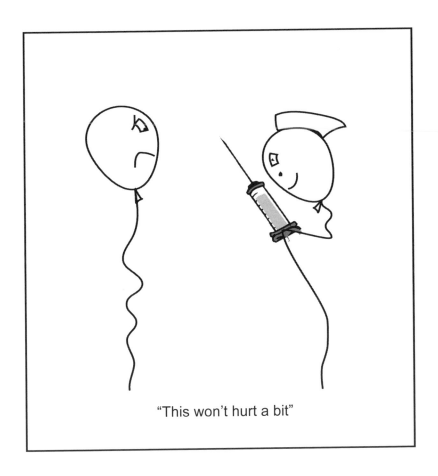

"This won't hurt a bit"

# 3.1.) <u>ABORTION (SPONTANEOUS)</u>

| | |
|---|---|
| **Risk factors** | ○ age < 15 years<br>○ age > 35 years<br>○ chromosomal abnormalities<br>○ endometritis<br>○ cervical incompetence |
| **Management** | **1.** karyotype aborted fetus for genetic abnormalities<br>**2.** consider cervical cerclage |

*Vaginal bleeding in early pregnancy is common and usually does not present spontaneous abortion.*

# 3.2.) <u>ABRUPTIO PLACENTAE</u>

| | |
|---|---|
| **Risk factors** | ○ cocaine, smoking<br>○ multiparity<br>○ hypertension |
| **Management** | **1.** replace fluids and blood vigorously<br>**2.** watch for signs of DIC |
| **Prognosis** | 1% maternal mortality<br>up to 50% fetal mortality |

# 3.3.) ACNE VULGARIS

| Risk factors | <ul><li>male</li><li>androgens</li><li>anabolic steroids</li><li>oily cosmetics</li></ul> |
|---|---|
| Management | 1. topical benzoyl peroxidase or tretinoin [1]<br>2. topical antibiotics<br>3. oral antibiotics or isotretinoin |

[1] *teratogenic! Do NOT use during pregnancy!*


# 3.4.) ACTINIC KERATOSIS

| Risk factors | <ul><li>fair skin</li><li>high elevation</li><li>sun exposure</li></ul> |
|---|---|
| Management | **Mild:** laser, cryo or other forms of dermabrasion<br>**Proliferative**: excision with margin<br><br>Advise patient to use sun protection! |
| Prognosis | 2~5% will progress to squamous cell carcinoma |

# 3.5.) <u>ACUTE RENAL FAILURE</u>

| | |
|---|---|
| **Risk factors** | ○ surgery<br>○ volume depletion<br>➤ aminoglycosides<br>➤ cyclosporine<br>➤ ACE inhibitors<br>➤ radio contrast |
| **Prevention** | • good hydration prior to contrast or chemotherapy<br>• aggressive restoration of intravascular volume |

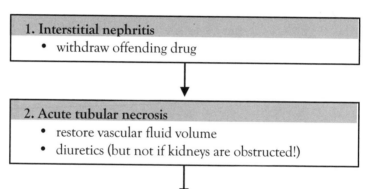

**1. Interstitial nephritis**
- withdraw offending drug

**2. Acute tubular necrosis**
- restore vascular fluid volume
- diuretics (but not if kidneys are obstructed!)

**3. Crescentic glomerulonephritis**
- diagnosis needs to be made by renal biopsy
- steroids
- cyclophosphamide

# 3.6.) ADDISON'S DISEASE
### Adrenal Insufficiency

| | |
|---|---|
| **Risk factors** | o  family history<br>o  prolonged intake of steroids<br>o  severe infection<br>o  severe trauma |
| **2° Prevention** | •  prevent adrenal crisis<br>•  daily hydrocortisone<br>•  double dose during illness or preoperative |
| **Management** | **Acute:**  hydrocortisone, IV<br>replace Na and glucose<br><br>**Chronic:**  oral hydrocortisone<br>patient should carry medic alert card |

# 3.7.) PRIMARY ALDOSTERONISM

**1. Unilateral adrenal adenoma**
- surgical removal → cure

↓

**2. Bilateral adenoma or zona glomerulosa hyperplasia**
- aldosterone antagonist (spironolactone)
- ACE inhibitor

# 3.8.) ALTITUDE SICKNESS

| Risk factors | o rapid ascent<br>o lack of conditioning |
|---|---|
| **Prevention** | • gradual ascent<br>• good hydration<br>➤ acetazolamide |
| **Management** | **1.** descend!!!<br>**2.** oxygen and/or hyperbaric bag<br>**3.** dexamethasone to reduce cerebral edema<br>**4.** nifedipine to reduce pulmonary distress |
| **Complications** | **Pulmonary edema** → respiratory distress syndrome<br>**Cerebral edema** → seizures, coma, death |

 *Patients may resume ascent if symptoms resolve.*


# 3.9.) ALZHEIMER'S DISEASE
### most common cause of dementia

| Risk factors | o age<br>o positive family history<br>o Down syndrome<br>o aberrant apolipoprotein (ApoE4) |
|---|---|
| **Management** | • Family support<br>  - adult day care, assisted living facilities<br><br>➤ CNS cholinesterase inhibitor: donepezil<br>➤ NMDA receptor antagonist if severe<br>➤ (Ginkgo biloba probably not helpful) |

142

# 3.10.) AMYLOIDOSIS

| Risk factors | **AL:** | multiple myeloma<br>other plasma cell disorders |
| --- | --- | --- |
| | **AA:** | chronic inflammatory diseases |
| Management | • control underlying chronic inflammation<br>• renal involvement may require kidney transplant | |

# 3.11.) AMYOTROPHIC LATERAL SCLEROSIS

| Risk factors | o age > 40 years<br>o positive family history |
| --- | --- |
| Management | **1.** physical therapy to maintain patient's independence<br>**2.** provide psychological counseling<br>**3.** Riluzole slows progression of disease<br>(inhibitor of presynaptic glutamate release)<br>**4.** Baclofen for muscle cramps |

# 3.12.) ANAPHYLACTIC SHOCK

| | |
|---|---|
| **Risk factors** | o  genetic predisposition <br> o  previous anaphylaxis |
| **Prevention** | •  avoid drugs/food that cause reaction <br> •  wear medical ID <br> •  advise to carry emergency epinephrine kit if patient has history of insect stings |

---

**1. If life-threatening:**

- initial CPR, $O_2$ , IV fluids
- epinephrine IM (repeat if necessary)

↓

**2. If not life-threatening, consider:**

- epinephrine
- antihistamines
- glucocorticoids

↓

**3. Monitor patient**

- late reactions possible 6~12 hours after acute event
- consult with allergist

 *Consider skin test prior to administration of high risk drugs.*

# 3.13.) ANKYLOSING SPONDYLITIS

| | |
|---|---|
| **Risk factors** | o  male gender<br>o  Caucasians<br>o  HLA-B27<br>o  inflammatory bowel disease |
| **Management** | **1.** physical exercises are extremely important<br>**2.** maintain good posture<br>**3.** NSAIDs: indomethacin<br>**4.** Disease modifying: sulfasalazine, methotrexate |

<u>Other diseases associated with HLA-B27</u>:
o  Reiter's syndrome
o  Uveitis
o  Juvenile rheumatoid arthritis
o  Psoriatic arthritis

# 3.14.) ANORECTAL ABSCESS

| | |
|---|---|
| **Risk factors** | o  prolapsed hemorrhoids<br>o  inflammatory bowel disease<br>o  previous perirectal abscess |
| **Prevention** | •  avoid constipation (fiber rich diet)<br>•  avoid enemas<br>•  perianal cleanliness |
| **Management** | •  incision and drainage!<br>(do not delay! do not "attempt antibiotics"!) |

# 3.15.) <u>ANOREXIA NERVOSA</u>

| | |
|---|---|
| **Risk factors** | ○ perfectionistic personality<br>○ high self-expectations<br>○ ambivalence about dependence / independence |
| **Management** | **1.** restore body weight and electrolytes<br>(best done under hospital supervision)<br>**2.** psychotherapy or family therapy |
| **Prognosis** | 50% will achieve normal weight<br>6% will die<br><br>→ early onset indicates better prognosis |

 *Rituals and abnormal attitudes towards food often persist.*

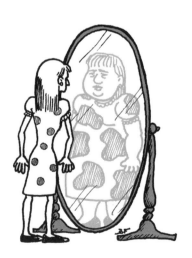

*"I look too fat..."*

# 3.16.) ANXIETY

| | |
|---|---|
| **Risk factors** | o family history<br>o lack of social support |
| **prevention** | • avoid stress<br>• relaxation techniques<br>• meditation |
| **Management** | • best results if antianxiety medication is combined with long-term psychotherapy |

# 3.17.) AORTIC DISSECTION

| | |
|---|---|
| **Risk factors** | o hypertension <br> o Marfan syndrome <br> o Ehlers-Danlos syndrome <br> o congenital aortic valve abnormalities <br> o coarctation of aorta <br> o trauma |
| **Prognosis** | 10-year survival after surgery 60% |

---

**1. Type A: ascending arch proximal to left subclavian a.**
- emergency surgery

↓

**2. Type B: descending aorta**
- medical management often sufficient
  β-blockers to reduce blood pressure
- surgery if distal ischemia develops

↓

**3. Follow-up**
- good control of hypertension is extremely important
- CT or MRI to detect developing aneurysms

# 3.18.) <u>AORTIC STENOSIS</u>

| Risk factors | **Young adults:** congenital<br>**Adults:** rheumatic<br>**Elderly:** calcification |
|---|---|
| 2° Prevention | • bacterial endocarditis prophylaxis<br>• rheumatic fever prophylaxis<br>• avoid exercise to prevent sudden death |
| Management | 1. replace valve before left ventricular dysfunction occurs<br>2. surgery is mandatory for symptomatic patients<br>3. balloon dilatation is effective, but may lead to aortic insufficiency |

*Aortic stenosis is the second most fatal heart valve disease after mitral regurgitation*

# 3.19.) <u>APLASTIC ANEMIA</u>

| Risk factors | **Hereditary**<br>  o Fanconi's anemia (autosomal recessive)<br>**Acquired**<br>  o viral illness<br>  o organic solvents<br>  ➤ chloramphenicol |
|---|---|
| Management | **if HLA-identical sibling available:**<br>• allogenic bone marrow transplant success rate is ~75%<br>**if no HLA-match is available:**<br>• immunosuppression |

# 3.20.) ARDS
## Acute Respiratory Distress Syndrome

Any injury to alveolar epithelium can result in ARDS:

| | |
|---|---|
| **Risk factors** | o  toxic inhalation<br>o  sepsis<br>o  shock<br>o  diffuse pneumonia |
| **Management** | **1.** identify the cause<br>**2.** mechanical ventilation<br>**3.** try to avoid barotrauma to the lungs<br>**4.** glucocorticoids for late phase ARDS<br>    (but not beneficial during acute stage) |
| **Prognosis** | 50~70% mortality |

 **PEEP** is used to increase oxygenation at a fixed $pO_2$.

# 3.21.) ARTERIAL THROMBOSIS/EMBOLUS

| | |
|---|---|
| **Risk factors** | **Embolus**<br>o atrial flutter/fibrillation<br><br>**Thrombosis**<br>o atherosclerosis<br>o aneurysm<br>o vascular injury |
| **Prevention** | • anticoagulation<br>• reduce risk factors for atherosclerosis |
| **Management** | 1. anticoagulation with IV heparin<br>2. consider TPA to dissolve thrombus<br>3. if limb is in jeopardy → revascularization surgery |

# 3.22.) ASPERGILLOSIS

| | |
|---|---|
| **Risk factors** | **Allergic:** exposure<br>**Aspergilloma:** pre-existing COPD, bronchiectasis, TB<br>**Systemic:** immunosuppression |
| **Prevention** | **Allergic:** avoid dead plants, compost piles…<br>**Aspergilloma:** treat underlying lung disease |
| **Management** | 1. voriconazole drug of choice for invasive aspergillosis<br>2. severe hemoptysis due to fungus ball may require surgery |

# 3.23.) <u>ASTHMA</u>

| | |
|---|---|
| **Risk factors** | ○ positive family history |
| **2° Prevention** | **Avoid triggering factors:**<br>• pollutants, dust, molds, <u>cold</u>, exercise<br><br>**Avoid aspirin** |

---

**1. Symptomatic relief:**
- β-2 agonists: albuterol, terbutaline
- xanthines: theophylline

↓

**2. Long-term control of disease:**
- cromolyn (mast cell stabilizer)
- inhaled glucocorticoid
- inhaled glucocorticoid plus bronchodilator

↓

**3. Status asthmaticus**
- hospitalization
- monitor arterial blood gases
- oxygen
- IV glucocorticoids

 *Find the minimum level of treatment to suppress symptoms and teach patient how to take responsibility for management of disease.*

# 3.24.) ATELECTASIS (POSTOPERATIVE)

| | |
|---|---|
| **Background** | • common in general anesthesia and ICU setting |
| **Risk factors** | ○ smoking<br>○ obesity |
| **Prevention** | • early postoperative mobilization<br>• aspiration precautions<br>• avoid 100% pure oxygen |
| **Management** | 1. provide adequate pain control in surgical patients<br>2. chest physiotherapy: percussion, drainage<br>3. nasotracheal suction to remove secretions<br>4. antibiotics for pneumonia or bronchitis |

# 3.25.) ATOPIC DERMATITIS

| | |
|---|---|
| **Risk factors** | ○ genetic predisposition<br>○ emotional stress |
| **3° Prevention** | • avoid aggravating factors:<br>(cold, soaps, detergents, other irritants…) |
| **Management** | 1. avoid drying of skin (soap, shampoos)<br>2. apply hydrophilic ointments (Eucerin) after bath or shower<br>3. tar shampoos reduce scalp itching<br>4. topical steroids (1% hydrocortisone) for inflamed areas |

# 3.26.) ATHEROSCLEROSIS
leading cause of mortality/morbidity in Western countries

| Risk factors | o hypertension<br>o high LDL, low HDL<br>o diabetes mellitus<br>o smoking<br>o obesity |
|---|---|
| Prevention | • reduce modifiable risk factors<br>• **diet:** < 30% of total calories from fat |

 *Lipid targets should be adjusted, depending on presence of other risk factors for cardiovascular disease!*

# 3.27.) ATRIAL FIBRILLATION

| Risk factors | o hypertension<br>o rheumatic heart disease<br>o left ventricular hypertrophy |
|---|---|
| Prevention | • long-term anticoagulation is required since atrial fibrillation recurs often despite anti-arrhythmics |
| Management | **Acute fibrillations:** - calcium channel blockers<br>- beta blockers<br>- digoxin<br><br>**Sustained fibrillations:** attempt cardioversion [1] |

[1] *Patient MUST be anticoagulated beforehand (risk of embolus)!*

# 3.28.) ATRIAL SEPTAL DEFECT

10% of congenital heart defects

| Risk factors | **Ostium primum defect:** Down syndrome<br>**Ostium secundum defect:** most cases sporadic |
| --- | --- |
| Management | **1.** small defects may be left unrepaired<br>**2.** surgical closure should be performed before<br>pulmonary hypertension develops! |
| Complications | • atrial fibrillation<br>• tricuspid regurgitation<br>• right sided heart failure |

# 3.29.) ADHD

**Attention Deficit Hyperactivity Disorder**

| Risk factors | o poor prenatal health |
| --- | --- |
| 3° Prevention | • support and advice to lessen risk for abuse,<br>depression, and social isolation |
| Management | **1.** assess parental involvement<br>**2.** behavioral intervention<br>**3.** consider Ritalin or dextroamphetamine<br>(start at lowest dose, observe effect) |

*Children with ADHD often develop antisocial personality
disorder later in life.*

# 3.30.) AUTISM

| Risk factors | o male<br>o paternal age<br>o genetic (high monozygotic twin concordance) |
|---|---|
| Management | • most patients need lifelong supervised care<br>(only 1~2% will become independent) |

# 3.31.) AUTOIMMUNE HEMOLYTIC ANEMIA

| Risk factors | **Warm antibodies IgG (90%)**<br>o "idiopathic"<br>o leukemia, lymphoma, myeloma<br>➤ drugs: methyldopa, quinidine….<br><br>**Cold antibodies IgM (10%)**<br>o "idiopathic"<br>o mycoplasma, mononucleosis |
|---|---|
| Management | 1. prednisone<br>2. blood transfusions: monitor very carefully<br>3. if renal impairment → aggressive hydration and<br>　　　　　　　　　　　　　　diuresis<br><br>4. search for underlying cause!<br><br>　- consider splenectomy<br>　- consider immunosuppression<br>　- Rituximab (antibody against B lymphocytes) |

*Cold agglutinin disease: prednisone and splenectomy are usually ineffective…*

# 3.32.) BASAL CELL CARCINOMA

| | |
|---|---|
| **Incidence** | 500,000 non-melanoma skin cancers/year in US (80% of these are BCC) |
| **Risk factors** | o sun exposure<br>o fair skin |
| **Prevention** | • sunscreen, hat… |
| **Prognosis** | • metastatic potential 0.1% |

*Non-melanotic skin cancer is the most common cancer in the US, but is usually excluded from cancer epidemiology tables because of its low fatality rate.*

# 3.33.) BENIGN PROSTATE HYPERPLASIA

| | |
|---|---|
| **Risk factors** | ➢ increased estradiol levels with age |
| **Management** | 1. digital rectal exam and PSA levels to rule out malignancy<br>2. consider herbal remedies<br>3. alpha blocker or 5α-reductase inhibitor<br>4. TURP: transurethral resection of the prostate |
| **Prognosis** | Many patients will improve or stabilize even without treatment! |

# 3.34.) BLADDER INJURY

| | |
|---|---|
| **Risk factors** | o blunt trauma to lower abdomen<br>o distended bladder at time of trauma<br>o prior pelvic surgery |
| **Prevention** | • wear seat belts |
| **Management** | 1. requires catheterization until hematuria resolves<br>2. rupture involving bladder neck → surgical repair<br>3. intraperitoneal ruptures → surgical repair |

# 3.35.) BOTULISM

| | |
|---|---|
| **Risk factors** | **Adults:** home-canned food<br>**Infants:** contaminated honey |
| **Prevention** | • no honey to infants < 12 months of age |
| **Management** | 1. support respiratory function<br>2. give *C. botulinum* antitoxin<br>  - contact CDC<br>  - make sure patient is not allergic to antitoxin |
| **Prognosis** | **Adults:** 10% mortality with intensive care<br>**Infants:** < 1% fatality rate if hospitalized |

# 3.36.) BRAIN ABSCESS

| Risk factors | o childhood poverty in developing countries<br>o immunosuppression<br>➢ IV drug abuse |
|---|---|
| Prevention | • early treatment of otitis media and dental abscesses<br>• prophylactic antibiotics after penetrating head wounds |
| Management | 1. be careful with lumbar puncture!<br>2. CSF → bacterial culture, antibiotic sensitivity<br>3. empirical antibiotic therapy<br>   - 3$^{rd}$ generation cephalosporin + metronidazole<br>4. consider dexamethasone to reduce edema |
| Prognosis | 10% mortality even with early detection (CT or MRI)<br>neurological sequelae in up to 50% |

# 3.37.) BREAST ABSCESS

| Risk factors | o puerperal mastitis<br>o nipple retraction |
|---|---|
| Prevention | • early treatment of mastitis<br>(milk expression, cold compresses, antibiotics) |
| Management | • nursing should be discontinued if abscess develops |

# 3.38.) BREAST CANCER

| | |
|---|---|
| **Background** | 1 in 8 women during lifetime |
| **Risk factors** | o  positive family history<br>o  early menarche<br>o  late menopause<br>o  nulliparity<br>o  (high dietary fat) |
| **2° Prevention** | **MAMMOGRAPHY:**<br>• every 1~2 years after 50 years of age<br>• annual clinical exam after 40 years of age |

**1. Stage I (tumor < 2cm, no axillary nodes)**
- lumpectomy with axillary lymph node resection
- *or* modified radical mastectomy
- consider adjuvant chemotherapy or hormonal therapy

**2. Stage II (tumor < 5cm or axillary node)**
- same options as stage I
- add radiation if several lymph nodes are involved

**3. Stage III (tumor > 5cm or chest wall extension)**
- preoperative chemotherapy
- followed by mastectomy

**4. Stage IV (metastatic)**
- chemotherapy / radiation / hormonal therapy
- biphosphonate to reduce bone metastases

# 3.39.) <u>BREECH BIRTH</u>

| | |
|---|---|
| **Risk factors** | o low birth weight, prematurity<br>o trisomy 21<br>o placenta previa |
| **Management** | • external version can be attempted at 30~36 weeks |

Normal position
(head first – occiput anterior)

Frank Breech presentation

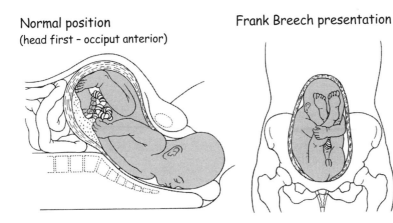

Full Breech presentation

Footling Breech presentation

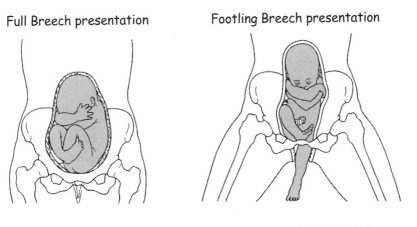

From *The Source Book of Medical Illustration*, 2nd edition, pp. 294-9, edited by P. Cull.

Copyright 1991 by Parthenon Publishing Group Limited, Lancaster, England.

# 3.40.) BRONCHIECTASIS

from chronic, recurrent bacterial infections

| | |
|---|---|
| **Risk factors** | ○ foreign body aspiration<br>○ chronic respiratory infection |
| **Prevention** | • immunization pneumonia/influenza<br>• treat pneumonia aggressively |
| **Management** | 1. 2~4 weeks antibiotics<br>(may have to try several different ones)<br>2. bronchodilators<br>3. percussion / postural drainage to clear secretions |

 *Less common nowadays thanks to antibiotics.*

# 3.41.) BRONCHIOLITIS

acute inflammation of small airways, usually caused by viruses

| | |
|---|---|
| **Risk factors** | ○ newborns (2~6 months)<br>○ day care environment |
| **Prevention** | • hand washing<br>• avoid contact with infected persons |
| **Management** | 1. correct hypoxemia if present<br>2. watch for dehydration due to tachypnea<br>3. consider ribavirin if due to RSV |

# 3.42.) BRUCELLOSIS

| Risk factors | o contact with cattle/sheep<br>o unpasteurized milk<br>o imported cheese |
|---|---|
| **Prevention** | • protective measures for meat and dairy workers<br>• avoid fresh milk |
| **Management** | ➤ Doxycycline + Rifampin<br>• watch out for relapse! |

# 3.43.) BURKITT'S LYMPHOMA
### highly aggressive NHL

| Risk factors | 90% of Burkitt's lymphoma in Africa a/w with EBV |
|---|---|
| **Management** | ➤ high-dose chemotherapy regimen |

# 3.44.) BURNS

## 1. Minor burns

- immediate cooling within 1$^{st}$ minute of burn decreases injury
- gentle débridement of loose tissue
- biologic dressing, sterile gauze
- apply topical antibiotic daily

## 2. Major burns

- if > 10~20% of body surface area → refer to burn center
- if burn involves face, hands or feet → refer to burn center

- replace fluids (Ringer's lactate)
- replace electrolytes (K$^+$, Ca$^{2+}$, Mg$^{2+}$, phosphate)
- replace albumin

- provide high caloric intake (if possible via GI tract)

## EXTENT:

> *Rule of 9: The body is divided into 11 areas, each representing 9% of surface.*

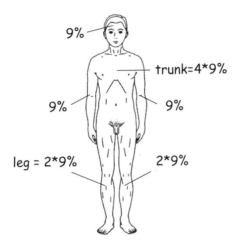

9%

trunk=4*9%

9%        9%

leg = 2*9%        2*9%

## DEGREE:

| First degree | - pink to red<br>- mild edema<br><br>- *no scarring* |
|---|---|
| **Second degree** | - pink to red, blanches on pressure<br>- blister formation<br>- hair does not pull out easily<br><br>- *scarring possible* |
| **Third degree** | - reddened areas don't blanch to pressure<br>- formation of devitalized, leathery tissue<br>- hair pulls out easily<br><br>- *scarring expected* |

## 3.45.) <u>SYSTEMIC CANDIDIASIS</u>

| | |
|---|---|
| **Risk factors** | ○ immunosuppression<br>○ mucocutaneous candidiasis |
| **Prevention** | • antibiotic prophylaxis for chemotherapy or bone marrow transplant patients |
| **Management** | ➢ fluconazole<br>➢ amphotericin B |

## 3.46.) <u>CONGENITAL CATARACT</u>

| | |
|---|---|
| **Risk factors** | ○ galactosemia<br>○ maternal diabetes<br>○ intrauterine infections (TORCH) [1]<br><br>➢ glucocorticoids [1]<br>➢ sulfonamides [1] |
| **Management** | **1.** surgical removal of lens material<br>**2.** contact lenses |

[1] *highest risk during first trimester*

 *In 50~60% of cases no cause can be identified.*

# 3.47.) CELIAC DISEASE

| | |
|---|---|
| **Risk factors** | o family history<br>o HLA-DR3 |
| **3° Prevention** | • gluten-free diet<br>(avoid wheat, barley, rye, oats) |
| **Management** | **1.** refer patient to dietitian<br>**2.** replace vitamins and minerals<br>**3.** 80% become symptom-free after several<br>weeks/months on strict gluten-free diet |

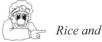 *Rice and corn are OK.*

# 3.48.) CEREBRAL PALSY

| | |
|---|---|
| **Risk factors** | o prematurity<br>o hypoxia<br>o perinatal seizures<br>o meningitis/encephalitis |
| **Management** | **1.** physical therapy<br>occupational therapy<br>speech training<br>**2.** should attend normal school if possible |

# 3.49.) CERVICAL CANCER

| Risk factors | o human papilloma virus (types 16, 18, 31, 33…)<br>o smoking |
|---|---|
| **Prevention** | • HPV vaccine |
| **2° Prevention** | • annual **Pap smear** for all sexually active women |

---

**1. Stage I (confined to cervix)**
- if fertility is desired: conization possible for Stage 1A
- modified radical hysterectomy
- if depth > 3mm → treat like stage II

↓

**2. Stage II (extends beyond cervix)**
- radical hysterectomy or radiation therapy
  (equally effective, cure rate ~98%)
- if parametrium is affected → treat like stage III

↓

**3. Stage III (extends to lower 1/3 of vagina)**
**4. Stage IV (extends beyond true pelvis)**
- radiation therapy
- plus chemotherapy

 *Do NOT combine surgery and radiation therapy!*

# 3.50.) CHANCROID

soft painful ulcers caused by *Haemophilus ducreyi*

| | |
|---|---|
| **Risk factors** | o multiple sexual partners<br>o uncircumcised males<br>o prostitutes |
| **Prevention** | • sexual counseling<br>• condoms<br>• treat partners |
| **Management** | ➢ ceftriaxone or ciprofloxacin |

# 3.51.) CHICKEN POX

| | |
|---|---|
| **Prevention** | • active immunization for children > 1 years<br>• passive immunization for immunocompromised who were exposed |
| **Management** | ➢ acetaminophen for fever<br>➢ antipruritic creams or ointments<br>➢ acyclovir for immunocompromised patients |
| **Complications** | • pneumonia<br>• encephalitis |

 *10% of adult population in US is susceptible.*

# 3.52.) CHLAMYDIA TRACHOMATIS

### most common STD in USA

| | |
|---|---|
| **Risk factors** | o lower socioeconomic groups<br>o sexual promiscuity |
| **Prevention** | • sexual counseling<br>• screen "target population" |
| **Management** | ➤ doxycycline (but not if pregnant!!!) |
| **Complications** | Chronic PID is very common due to asymptomatic nature of the disease and non-compliance with treatment. |

*Most women are asymptomatic for months or years!*
*Treat partners (if you can find them).*

# 3.53.) CHOLECYSTITIS

| Background | 50% of patients with gallstones will develop symptoms |
|---|---|
| Risk factors | o cholelithiasis <br> o biliary parasites |
| Management | **1.** NSAIDS <br> **2.** laparoscopic cholecystectomy |

# 3.54.) CHOLELITHIASIS

| Risk factors | o female <br> o multiparity <br> o obesity <br> o rapid weight loss |
|---|---|
| Management | **1.** in most cases, removal of asymptomatic gallbladder is NOT recommended <br> **2.** attempt dissolution if asymptomatic (ursodeoxycholic acid) |
| Prognosis | 1~2% of patients per year will develop symptoms requiring surgery |

**1. Acute cholecystitis**
- broad-spectrum antibiotic
- place patient on NPO
- surgery after 24~48 hours

**2. Chronic cholecystitis**
- elective laparoscopic cholecystectomy

# 3.55.) CHOLERA

| | |
|---|---|
| **Risk factors** | o travel to epidemic areas<br>o contaminated food, water |
| **Prevention** | • water purification<br>• no unpeeled raw fruits/vegetables<br>➤ tetracycline for contacts<br>➤ prophylactic vaccine is NOT recommended |
| **Management** | **1.** Oral rehydration solution (water + salt + sugar)<br>to replace fluid and electrolytes lost with stool<br>**2.** tetracycline/doxycycline |
| **Prognosis** | mortality < 1% if treated with ORS |

# 3.56.) CLUSTER HEADACHE

Attacks occur in "cluster" cycles, lasting weeks or months with almost daily attacks.

| | |
|---|---|
| **Risk factors** | o male<br>o age > 30 years<br>➤ vasodilators |
| **Prophylaxis**<br>(during cluster cycle) | ➤ lithium<br>➤ ergotamine at bedtime<br>• avoid alcohol |
| **Acute attack**<br>(teatment is difficult) | **1.** sumatriptan<br>**2.** 100% $O_2$ by mask<br>**3.** try methysergide or glucocorticoid |

# 3.57.) CMV INFECTION

most common congenital infection in developed countries

| Risk factors | o  organ transplantation<br>o  immunosuppression<br>o  AIDS |
|---|---|
| **Prevention** | •  if patient is seronegative for CMV, try to avoid transplanting from CMV positive donor |
| **Management** | ➤  ganciclovir for disseminated infection / retinitis |
| **Prognosis** | major cause of morbidity in organ transplant patients (especially bone marrow transplants) |

 *Risk of intrauterine infection 50~100% when primary maternal infection happens during pregnancy.*


# 3.58.) COARCTATION OF AORTA

| Risk factors | o  other congenital heart abnormalities<br>o  Turner's syndrome |
|---|---|
| **Management** | •  resection of narrowed segment (10-year survival after surgery > 90%) |

# 3.59.) <u>*COCCIDIOIDOMYCOSIS*</u>

| | |
|---|---|
| **Risk factors** | o endemic to Southwest of US<br>o lab cultures are highly contagious!<br><br>o high risk of disseminated disease in AIDS |
| **Prevention** | • avoid exposure (especially high risk population) |
| **Management** | **1.** if uncomplicated → observe<br>**2.** if pulmonary or disseminated  disease → itraconazole |

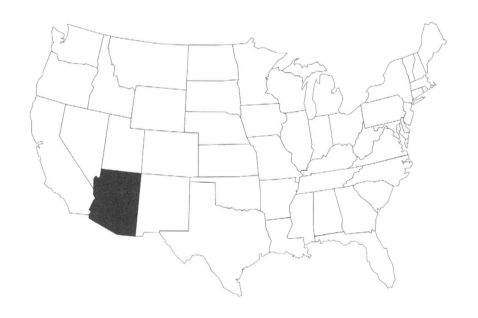

 *If disseminated → high mortality!*

# 3.60.) COLORECTAL CANCER

| | |
|---|---|
| **Risk factors** | o ulcerative colitis<br>o familial polyposis<br>o adenomatous polyps<br><br>o high dietary animal fat<br>o low dietary fiber intake |
| **Management** | **COLON CANCER**<br>**1.** surgical resection<br>**2.** resection plus chemotherapy for Duke C<br>**3.** postoperative screening: CEA<br>    endoscopy 1 year post-op, then regular schedule<br><br>**RECTAL CANCER**<br>**1.** preoperative radiotherapy improves survival |
| **Prognosis** | |

|  |  | **5-year survival** |
|---|---|---|
| **Stage I** | (mucosa and submucosa) | > 90% |
| **Stage II** | (through serosa) | 50~90% |
| **Stage III** | (regional lymph nodes) | 20~50% |
| **Stage VI** | (distant metastases) | < 5% |

# 3.61.) CONSTIPATION

| Risk factors | ○ sedentary lifestyle<br>➢ drugs: anticholinergics |
|---|---|
| Management | **1.** high fiber diet (recommend 20~30 g/day)<br>**2.** increase fluid intake<br><br>**3.** laxatives:   bulk      (Metamucil)<br>                 osmotic   (Magnesium)<br>                 stimulant  (Senna) |

# 3.62.) CONTACT DERMATITIS

| Risk factors | ○ cosmetics<br>○ jewelry<br>○ occupational exposure |
|---|---|
| Management | **1.** avoid exposure<br>**2.** use gloves with cotton lining |

# 3.63.) COPD

| | |
|---|---|
| **Risk factors** | ○ smoking<br>○ passive smoking, air pollution<br>○ viral pneumonia in early life<br>○ airway hyperreactivity<br>○ $\alpha$1-antitrypsin deficiency |
| **Prevention** | • stop smoking<br>• vaccinate against pneumonia and influenza |
| **Management** | **1.** symptomatic relief<br>  • anticholinergic bronchodilators<br>    - if required add $\beta$2-agonist<br>  • glucocorticoids for acute inflammation<br>  • broad-spectrum antibiotics<br>**2.** supplemental home $O_2$ reduces mortality<br>**3.** late stage → consider lung volume reduction surgery<br><br>• monitor lung function ($FEV_1$)<br>• annual chest X-ray |

*COPD with predominant bronchitis has better prognosis than with predominant emphysema.*

# 3.64.) <u>CORONARY ARTERY DISEASE</u>
### causes 1/3 of deaths in US (myocardial infarction)

| | |
|---|---|
| **Risk factors** | o  male<br>o  hypertension<br>o  diabetes mellitus<br>o  high LDL<br>o  low HDL<br>o  smoking<br>o  obesity |
| **Management** | **1.** recommend low fat/low cholesterol diet<br>**2.** promote smoking cessation<br>**3.** control blood pressure<br>**4.** consider prophylactic aspirin<br>**5.** estrogen replacement in postmenopausal women |
| **Prognosis** | **<u>Risk of myocardial infarction</u>**<br>• The relative risk of smokers approaches that of non-smokers within 2~3 years of smoking cessation.<br><br>• 1% decrease in serum cholesterol lowers risk by 2~3%<br>• 1 mmHg decrease in blood pressure lowers risk 2~3%<br>• maintaining active lifestyle lowers risk by 45% |

*Treadmill stress test is NOT recommended as routine screening for adults with no evidence of coronary heart disease.*

---

### <u>Dietary Goals To Prevent Heart Disease:</u>

Less than 2 risk factors:     LDL <160 mg/dL
2 or more risk factors:     LDL <130 mg/dL
Coronary heart disease:     LDL <100 mg/dL

## CORONARY ARTERIES:

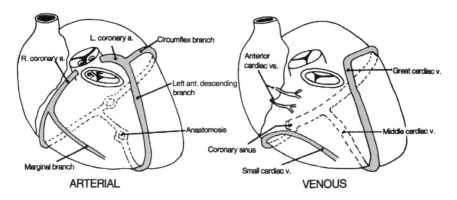

From Goldberg: *Clinical Anatomy Made Ridiculously Simple*, MedMaster, 2007

# 3.65.) COR PULMONALE

| | |
|---|---|
| **Risk factors** | o living at high altitude<br>o smoking |
| **Prevention** | • stop smoking |
| **Prognosis** | COPD with cor pulmonale: 50% mortality in 3 years |

# 3.66.) CROHN'S DISEASE

| | |
|---|---|
| **Risk factors** | o Caucasians<br>o Jewish ancestry<br>o family history<br><br>o major psychological stress = trigger |
| **Prognosis** | - worse than ulcerative colitis<br>- mortality increases with duration of disease |

---

**1. Mild to moderate disease**
- sulfasalazine (more effective for colon than small bowels)
- antibiotics

↓

**2. Severe disease**
- Acute attack: glucocorticoids
  (should be tapered as soon as remission occurs)
- mercaptopurine or azathioprine to sustain remission
- experimental: antibodies to tumor necrosis factor!
- unresponsive, or obstructions → surgery

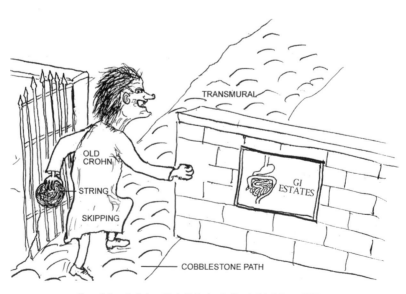

From Zaher: *Pathology Made Ridiculously Simple*, MedMaster, 2007

# 3.67.) CRYPTOCOCCOSIS

| Risk factors | ➤ immunosuppression<br>- reactivation of latent lung foci → pneumonia<br>- dissemination, meningitis |
|---|---|
| Prevention | • avoid pigeon droppings<br>➤ itraconazole prophylaxis for AIDS patients |
| Management | ➤ itraconazole |

# 3.68.) CRYPTORCHIDISM

| Risk factors | o prematurity<br>o family history |
|---|---|
| Management | **1.** try hCG to promote testicular descent<br>**2.** surgery (orchiopexy) at age of 6 months<br>**3.** orchiectomy if discovered post puberty |
| Prognosis | decreased fertility rate<br>10~50 fold increased risk of seminoma |

 *Orchiopexy does NOT reduce risk of malignant degeneration but facilitates early detection.*

# 3.69.) CUSHING'S SYNDROME

| | |
|---|---|
| **Causes** | **most common cause:** iatrogenic<br>**other causes:** 80% pituitary<br>20% adrenal |
| **Risk factors** | ➤ prolonged use of glucocorticoids |
| **Management** | **1.** transphenoidal removal of pituitary adenoma<br>**2.** if this fails, consider bilateral adrenalectomy<br>**3.** lifelong mineralocorticoid and glucocorticoid replacement after total adrenalectomy |

# 3.70.) CUTANEOUS DRUG REACTIONS

| | |
|---|---|
| **Risk factors** | ➤ penicillin, sulfonamides, many more… |
| **Prevention** | **Beware of likely crossover sensitivity:**<br>penicillin ↔ cephalosporins<br>hydantoin ↔ carbamazepine ↔ barbiturates |
| **Management** | **1.** topical antipruritics<br>**2.** antihistamines<br>**3.** systemic glucocorticoids for severe cases |

# 3.71.) CYSTIC FIBROSIS

most common lethal genetic disease in Caucasians

| Risk factors | o family history<br>o Ashkenazi Jews |
|---|---|
| Management | 1. daily chest physical therapy (percussion)<br>2. annual influenza immunization<br>3. avoid general anesthesia |
| Prognosis | average life expectancy now ~35 years |

# 3.72.) DEEP VEIN THROMBOSIS

| Risk factors | o prolonged immobility<br>o pregnancy<br>o oral contraceptives<br>o malignancies |
|---|---|
| Prevention | ➢ low-dose heparin<br>➢ low-dose warfarin<br>• compression stockings<br>• low estrogen content birth control pills |
| Management | 1. initial anticoagulation with heparin (monitor APTT)<br>2. oral anticoagulation with warfarin (monitor INR: 2~3)<br>for 3~6 months after acute event<br>3. if anticoagulation is contraindicated: vena cava filter |
| Prognosis | 20% of untreated DVT develop pulmonary embolism<br>(of these ~10% are fatal) |

# 3.73.) <u>DEMENTIA</u>

| | |
|---|---|
| **Risk factors** | o age<br>o family history<br>o atherosclerosis<br>o head trauma, CNS infection |
| **Management** | **1.** safety first: avoid alcohol, driving, etc.<br>**2.** wear medic alert card<br><br>*Ginkgo biloba* probably not effective |
| **Prognosis** | **Alzheimer type:**    always progressive<br><br>**Multi-infarct type:**    step-like<br>not always progressive |

# 3.74.) DIABETES MELLITUS TYPE 1
## IDDM

**Risk factors**

- o HLA-DR3
- o HLA-DR4
- o monozygotic twin concordance only 50%

---

### 1. Insulin
- morning dose before breakfast
- evening dose before dinner
- mix intermediate (NPH) with short acting (regular) insulins

### 2. Family education is extremely important!
- carbohydrate counting, <u>regular</u> meal times
- physical exercise: reduce insulin or provide extra snack

### 3. Follow-up
- quarterly physical exam, including $HBA_{1C}$

---

***Honeymoon effect:*** *Initial treatment with insulin restores some β-cell function → risk of hypoglycemia due to increased endogenous insulin.*

***Dawn phenomenon:*** *Early morning rise in glucose due to circadian changes in GH and cortisol.*

***Somogyi effect:*** *Exaggerated dawn phenomenon. Nocturnal hypoglycemia results in overshooting morning hyperglycemia. Manage by decreasing evening insulin.*

## 3.75.) <u>DIABETES MELLITUS TYPE 2</u>
### NIDDM

| Prevalence | 8% of US population and rising! |
|---|---|
| Risk factors | o gestational diabetes<br>o monozygotic twin concordance almost 100% |
| Prevention | • avoid obesity<br>• exercise |
| Management | **1.** sulfonylureas (short acting ones are safer)<br>**2.** metformin decreases hepatic gluconeogenesis<br>**3.** insulin often required for endstage type 2 diabetes |

 *>10% of US population has impaired glucose tolerance, but only some progress to overt diabetes mellitus.*

## 3.76.) <u>DIABETIC HYPOGLYCEMIA</u>

| Background | more common in type 1 diabetes |
|---|---|
| Risk factors | o gastroenteritis<br>o more common in tightly controlled patients treated for several years |
| Prevention | • patient education<br>• routine schedule/diet |
| Management | **1.** oral glucose (fruit juice)<br>**2.** if unable to take oral: glucagon<br>**3.** if comatose: IV glucose |

# 3.77.) DIABETIC KETOACIDOSIS

| Background | more common in type 1 diabetes |
|---|---|
| Risk factors | o physical or emotional stress<br>o trauma<br>o infections<br>o vomiting |
| Prevention | • monitor glucose during stressful situations |
| Management | 1. fluid replacement (0.9% saline)<br>2. insulin infusion (monitor glucose)<br>3. monitor $K^+$ hourly → add to infusion when $K^+$ starts to drop due to redistribution<br>4. bicarbonate for severe acidosis (pH<7) |

*Hyperosmolar coma* is more common than diabetic ketoacidosis in adults and elderly with type 2 diabetes.

# 3.78.) DIABETIC RETINOPATHY
leading cause of blindness in US

| Risk factors | o duration of diabetes mellitus<br>o poor glucose control<br>o systemic hypertension |
|---|---|
| Prevention | • tight control of blood glucose (monitor $HbA_{1C}$)<br>• aggressive treatment of hypertension |

# 3.79.) DIPHTHERIA

| Risk factors | o inadequate immunization<br>o minority racial groups |
|---|---|
| Prevention | **Immunization:**<br>• DTaP at 2,4,6 and 15 months<br>• booster every 10 years |
| Management | **1.** hospitalize (ICU)<br>**2.** give antitoxin<br>    - don't wait for bacterial culture!<br>    - monitor closely for hypersensitivity reaction!<br>**3.** penicillin |

*DTaP = Diphtheria, Tetanus, acellular Pertussis*


# 3.80.) DISCOID LUPUS ERYTHEMATOSUS

| Risk factors | o female<br>o African American<br>o systemic lupus erythematosus |
|---|---|
| Management | **1.** avoid sun exposure<br>**2.** avoid excessive heat or cold<br>**3.** avoid skin trauma |

# 3.81.) DISSOCIATIVE DISORDERS

> Dissociative amnesia: memory gaps from minutes to days.
> Fugue: patient assumes new name, identity and behavior but may appear normal.
> Identity disorder: multiple personalities alternate and "take over" patient's behavior.
> Depersonalization disorder: feeling of being detached from self.

| Risk factors | o neglect, abuse, trauma during childhood |
|---|---|
| Prevention | • child abuse prevention<br>• crisis intervention |
| Management | • supportive, stable environment<br>• psychotherapy<br>- consider hypnosis for identity disorder<br>• consider antianxiety medication |

# 3.82.) DIVERTICULOSIS

| Prevalence | 20~50% of US population over 50 years |
|---|---|
| Risk factors | o age<br>o low fiber diet |
| Management | **Diverticulosis**<br>• high fiber diet (20~30g/day)<br>➢ bulk forming laxatives (psyllium, methylcellulose)<br>• if bleeding → sigmoidoscopy, angiography<br><br>**Diverticulitis**<br>➢ antibiotics, bowel rest<br>➢ signs of peritonitis → hospitalize, IV antibiotics<br>• may require surgery |

# 3.83.) DROWNING

| | |
|---|---|
| **Risk factors** | o alcohol<br>o inadequate supervision of children |
| **Management** | **1.** hypothermia slows metabolism → always attempt resuscitation, even if patient was submerged long time<br>**2.** don't waste time trying to remove water from lungs<br>**3.** begin mouth-mouth and cardiac compression<br>**4.** if diving accident: suspect neck injury and stabilize<br>**5.** hospitalize, even if patient seems to recover! |

---

### MOST COMMON CAUSES OF ACCIDENTS:
#1 - motor vehicle accidents
#2 - falls
#3 - poisoning
#4 - burns
#5 – drowning

---

# 3.84.) DYSMENORRHEA

| | |
|---|---|
| **Prevalence** | 40% of adult females have menstrual pain<br>10% are incapacitated for a few days each month |
| **Risk factors** | **Primary dysmenorrhea**<br>o nulliparity<br>**Secondary dysmenorrhea**<br>o endometriosis<br>o pelvic infection<br>o STDs |
| **Prevention** | • reduce risk of STDs → secondary dysmenorrhea |
| **Management** | **1.** NSAIDs<br>**2.** daily calcium supplement<br>**3.** oral contraceptives<br>**4.** antidepressant (fluoxetine) during luteal phase |

# 3.85.) DYSPAREUNIA

| | |
|---|---|
| **Prevalence** | 1~2% of adult females |
| **Risk factors** | o endometriosis<br>o diabetes mellitus<br>o estrogen deficiency<br>o menopause |
| **Management** | **1.** examine both partners<br>**2.** provide counseling in sex techniques<br>   suggest non-penetrating sex<br>**3.** lidocaine cream |

# 3.86.) DYSPEPSIA
pain, discomfort in upper abdomen

| | |
|---|---|
| **Risk factors** | o anxiety<br>o depression<br>o other functional disorders |
| **Management** | **1.** frequent small meals<br>**2.** avoid:<br>   - coffee and tea<br>   - chocolate<br>   - alcohol and smoking<br>   - NSAIDs<br>**3.** search for underlying cause:<br>   - esophageal reflux<br>   - peptic ulcer disease<br>   - *H. pylori* infection |

 *Functional dyspepsia is a diagnosis of exclusion!*

# 3.87.) ECLAMPSIA

| | |
|---|---|
| **Risk factors** | o  primigravida<br>o  twin gestation<br>o  hydatidiform mole<br>o  preexisting renal disease or hypertension |
| **HELLP** | **Hepatic injury due to preeclampsia:**<br>•  **H**emolysis<br>•  **E**levated **L**iver enzymes<br>•  **L**ow **P**latelets |
| **Prognosis** | •  most cases of preeclampsia are mild<br>•  severe preeclampsia often due to preexisting renal disease or autoimmune disorders |

### 1. Preeclampsia
- bed rest
- hospitalization improves outcome
- control of preexisting hypertension
- monitor fetus: corticosteroids to accelerate lung maturation

↓

### 2. Eclampsia
- place patient in lateral position
- $Mg^{2+}$ sulfate IV for convulsions
- monitor fetal viability
- as soon as mother is stabilized → delivery

*Hypertension developing during pregnancy increases the likelihood of later "essential" hypertension.*

# 3.88.) ECTOPIC PREGNANCY

most common cause of maternal death in first half of pregnancy in US

| | |
|---|---|
| **Risk factors** | o pelvic inflammatory disease<br>o use of IUD<br>o endometritis<br>➤ "morning after pill" |
| **Prevention** | • ultrasound to verify location of pregnancy and to prevent complications of ectopic pregnancy (tubal rupture) |
| **Management** | **1.** if early → methotrexate (DNA synthesis inhibitor)<br>**2.** if late → laparoscopic surgery<br>**3.** follow-up: β-hCG levels |

# 3.89.) ENCEPHALITIS - VIRAL

| Risk factors | **Winter:** Mumps, Varicella<br>**Summer:** Arthropod-borne viruses<br>**Summer/Fall:** Enteroviruses |
|---|---|
| Management | 1. examine CSF for diagnosis<br>2. consider PCR of CSF to detect viral DNA or RNA<br>3. Acyclovir for herpes encephalitis<br>   Foscarnet: wide-spectrum anti-viral |
| Prognosis | neurologic sequelae in 10~80% depending on virus<br><br>**Worst prognosis:** EEE and herpes simplex [1] |

[1] *Herpes encephalitis is treatable! Early diagnosis is crucial!*

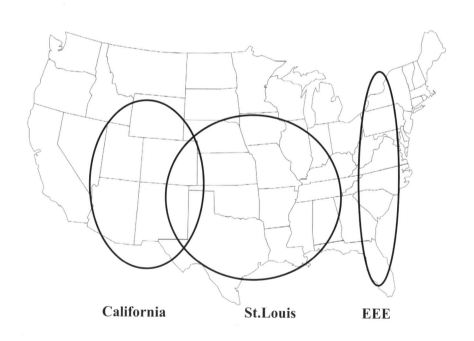

California          St.Louis          EEE

# 3.90.) ENDOCARDITIS (bacterial)

| | |
|---|---|
| **Risk factors** | o IV catheters<br>o IV drug abuse<br>o artificial valves<br>o acquired valve dysfunction |
| **Prevention** | • maintain good oral hygiene<br>• antibiotic prophylaxis prior to dental procedures |
| **Management** | **1.** empirical antibiotics (vancomycin + ceftriaxone)<br>against staphylo-, strepto- and enterococci<br>**2.** don't wait for result of culture! |

# 3.91.) ENDOMETRIAL CARCINOMA
most common gynecologic malignancy

| | |
|---|---|
| **Risk factors** | o age > 40 years<br>o early menarche<br>o late menopause<br>o nulliparity<br>o obesity |
| **Prevention** | ➢ avoid unopposed estrogen |

---

**1. Stage I (limited to endometrium)**
**2. Stage II (extends to cervix)**
• hysterectomy and bilateral salpingo-oophorectomy

**3. Stage III (confined to true pelvis)**
**4. Stage IV (invading bladder/rectum)**
• as above, plus add radiotherapy or chemotherapy
• consider hormonal therapy (progesterone)

# 3.92.) ENDOMETRIOSIS

| | |
|---|---|
| **Prevalence** | 10% of women of reproductive age |
| **Prevention** | • pregnancy may have positive effect |
| **Management** | **1.** hormone therapy:<br>- oral contraceptives<br>- induce amenorrhea → progesterone<br>                                 danazol<br>**2.** surgery:<br>- laparoscopic removal of lesions |

# 3.93.) ENURESIS

| | |
|---|---|
| **Prevalence** | 10% of children |
| **Risk factors** | ○ male<br>○ first born child<br>○ family history |
| **Management** | **1.** wetting alarms<br>**2.** drugs:<br>- desmopressin nasal spray<br>- imipramine |

# 3.94.) EPIGLOTTITIS

| Background | dramatically decreased since *H. influenzae* vaccine |
|---|---|
| Risk factors | o children 2~4 years |
| Management | 1. Hospitalize! IV antibiotics<br>2. Intubation may be necessary for 24~48 hours<br>3. Rifampin for household and day care contacts |

 *This is a medical emergency!*


# 3.95.) EPILEPSY

---

**1. Pharmacotherapy**
- "start low, go slow"
- may have to try several drugs
- only after 2 seizure-free years may drugs be withdrawn careful: taper off slowly

| ➤ Partial seizures: | carbamazepine, phenytoin |
|---|---|
| ➤ Generalized seizures: | valproic acid |
| ➤ Absence seizures: | ethosuximide |

↓

**2. Pregnancy**
- usually, the risk of discontinuing medication is larger than the risk of fetal abnormalities due to drug.

↓

**3. Status epilepticus**
- keep airways open
- lorazepam IV
- if seizures do not stop may require general anesthesia

---

# 3.96.) ERYSIPELAS

caused by group A beta-hemolytic streptococci

| | |
|---|---|
| **Risk factors** | o skin lesions, abrasions<br>o stasis dermatitis<br>o diabetes<br>o immunosuppression |
| **Management** | ➤ penicillin<br>• if recurrent, search for source of streptococcal infection |

# 3.97.) ERYTHEMA INFECTIOSUM

"Fifth disease" - Human parvovirus B19

| | |
|---|---|
| **Prevention** | • standard hygiene practices<br>• contagious period is before rash appears |
| **Management** | • symptomatic treatment of headache and fever |
| **Complications** | • risk of intrauterine infection<br>• risk of aplastic crisis in sickle cell patients |

 *Pregnant women should avoid patients with aplastic crisis.*

# 3.98.) ERYTHROBLASTOSIS FETALIS

| | |
|---|---|
| **Background** | most cases now due to ABO incompatibility<br>most <u>severe</u> cases still due to Rh incompatibility |
| **Risk factors** | o  Rh-positive fetus in Rh-negative woman<br>o  prior transfusion of incompatible blood<br><br>*Risk of sensitization without prophylaxis about 10%.* |
| **Prevention** | **1.** RhoGAM at 28~32 weeks for unsensitized women<br>(i.e. negative indirect Coombs test)<br>**2.** postpartum RhoGAM if baby is Rh-positive |

**1. Maternal management**
- monitor Rh antibody titers in Rh negative women
- if sensitized, perform amniocentesis → bilirubin

↓

**2. Fetal management**
- consider intravascular blood transfusion
  (into umbilical vein)
- glucocorticoids to accelerate fetal lung maturation
- deliver early (28 weeks)

↓

**3. Neonatal management**
- assess hematocrit and bilirubin levels
- phototherapy to avoid kernicterus

# 3.99.) ESOPHAGEAL CANCER

| | |
|---|---|
| **Risk factors** | **Squamous cell carcinoma (most common worldwide)**<br>o smoking<br>o alcohol<br><br>**Adenocarcinoma (most common in US)**<br>o Barrett's metaplasia |
| **Prevention** | • stop smoking<br>• limit alcohol |
| **Management** | **1.** if early and limited to mucosa → surgical resection<br>**2.** if advanced → chemotherapy or radiation<br>               followed by surgery |
| **Prognosis** | 5-year survival 5~10% |

# 3.100.) FALLOT'S TETRALOGY

> (1.) Ventricular septal defect
> (2.) Overriding aorta
> (3.) Pulmonary stenosis
> (4.) → Right ventricular hypertrophy

| | |
|---|---|
| **Background** | most common cyanotic heart disease after age 1 year |
| **Management** | • fatal unless surgically corrected |

## A) Transposition of Great Arteries

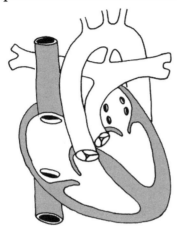

From Goldberg: *Clinical Anatomy Made Ridiculously Simple*, MedMaster, 2007

## B) Tetralogy of Fallot

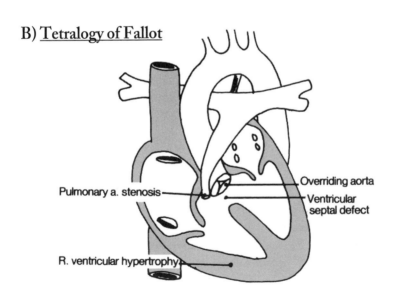

Pulmonary a. stenosis

Overriding aorta

Ventricular septal defect

R. ventricular hypertrophy

From Goldberg: *Clinical Anatomy Made Ridiculously Simple*, MedMaster, 2007

# 3.101.) <u>FEBRILE SEIZURES</u>

| | |
|---|---|
| **Prevalence** | 3~5% of children have one febrile seizure before age 5 |
| **Management** | **1.** acetaminophen prophylaxis during fever<br>**2.** diazepam prophylaxis <u>during high fever</u><br><br>continuous prophylaxis is controversial |
| **Prognosis** | • 70% one episode only<br>• most recurrences within 1 year<br>• risk of later epilepsy only 1~2% |

*Infants < 18 months do not have reliable signs of meningitis.
Consider lumbar puncture!*


# 3.102.) <u>FIBROCYSTIC CHANGE</u>

*This is NOT a disease. The term "fibrocystic breast disease"
should be avoided.*

| | |
|---|---|
| **Prevalence** | > 50% of adult women |
| **Prevention** | avoiding caffeine may reduce breast pain |
| **Prognosis** | no increase in cancer risk |

---

<u>RELATIVE RISK FOR BREAST CANCER</u>:

| | |
|---|---|
| **No increased cancer risk:** | fibrosis<br>fibroadenoma<br>mastitis<br>squamous metaplasia |
| **1.5~2fold cancer risk:** | florid adenosis<br>hyperplasia |
| **5fold cancer risk:** | atypical hyperplasia |

# 3.103.) FOOD ALLERGY

| | |
|---|---|
| **Prevalence** | 1~2% of adults, more common in children |
| **Risk factors** | ○ atopic predisposition |
| **Management** | • avoid offending food |
| **Prognosis** | **Infants:** usually outgrow their hypersensitivity<br>**Adults:** allergy often persists |

*"Perceived" food allergy is much more common than "true" food allergy.*


# 3.104.) FRAGILE-X SYNDROME
### second most common genetic cause of mental retardation
### (after Down syndrome)

| | |
|---|---|
| **Risk factors** | ○ fragile site on long arm of chromosome X |
| **Prevention** | • genetic counseling<br>(X-linked recessive disorder)<br>• consider amniocentesis |
| **Prognosis** | **Males:** mild to moderate retardation<br>**Females:** lower expression of disease than males |

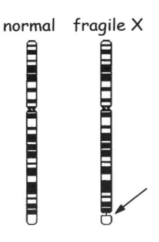

normal    fragile X

# 3.105.) GANGRENE

| Risk factors | o arteriosclerosis<br>o diabetes mellitus<br>o smoking<br>o trauma |
|---|---|
| Prevention | • good skin care<br>• avoid trauma |
| Management | 1. reduce risk factors for atherosclerosis!<br>2. regular exercise for patients with claudication<br>3. get surgical consultation → revascularization |

# 3.106.) GASTRIC ADENOCARCINOMA

| Incidence | dramatic decrease world wide |
|---|---|
| Risk factors | o pickled, salted, spicy Asian food<br>o food nitrates<br>o smoking<br>o polyposis |
| 2° Prevention | • Endoscopic screening in endemic areas (Japan) |
| Management | 1. early disease<br>   - resection<br>   - adjuvant chemotherapy is investigational<br>2. late disease<br>   - chemotherapy<br>   - surgery of palliative value only |

 *Gastric Lymphoma (MALT) has also been linked to H. pylori and has a much better prognosis than adenocarcinoma.*

# 3.107.) CHRONIC GASTRITIS TYPE A

### affects mostly corpus

| | |
|---|---|
| **Background** | much less common than type B chronic gastritis |
| **Risk factors** | ○ antibodies to parietal cells<br>○ antibodies to intrinsic factor |
| **Management** | • lifelong parenteral Vit. B12 prevents pernicious anemia |

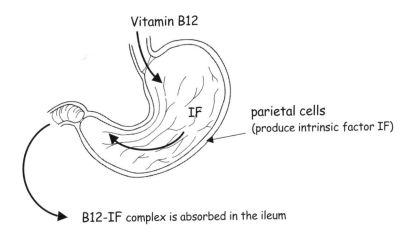

Vitamin B12

IF

parietal cells
(produce intrinsic factor IF)

B12-IF complex is absorbed in the ileum

# 3.108.) CHRONIC GASTRITIS TYPE B

### affects mostly antrum

| | |
|---|---|
| **Background** | 30~50% of population have chronic *H.pylori* infection. Most are asymptomatic! |
| **Risk factors** | o *H. pylori* infection |
| **Management** | PPI + sucralfate<br><br>***H.Pylori* "Triple Therapy"**<br>**1.** proton pump inhibitor (PPI)<br>**2.** plus clarithromycin<br>**3.** plus amoxicillin (or metronidazole) |
| **Prognosis** | • increased risk of gastric cancer<br>• increased risk of lymphoma (MALT) |

# 3.109.) EROSIVE GASTRITIS

| | |
|---|---|
| **Risk factors** | o shock<br>o burns<br>o sepsis<br>o trauma |
| **Management** | **ICU patients:** antacids or H$_2$-blockers<br>**NSAID users:** misoprostol |

*Overt bleeding from erosive gastritis in an ICU setting has a high mortality!*

# 3.110.) GASTROESOPHAGEAL REFLUX DISEASE

| | |
|---|---|
| **Risk factors** | **Foods that lower LES pressure:**<br>o chocolate, mint<br><br>**Irritant foods:**<br>o lemon juice, spicy tomato juice<br><br>**Other:**<br>o smoking, alcohol, coffee |
| **Management** | **1.** diet modification<br>**2.** antacids: proton pump inhibitors<br><br>**3.** annual endoscopy in patients with Barrett's metaplasia |

# 3.111.) GIARDIASIS

most common cause of water-borne gastroenteritis in US

| | |
|---|---|
| **Risk factors** | o camping<br>o day care centers<br>o male homosexuality |
| **Prevention** | • hand washing<br>• water purification/boiling when camping |
| **Management** | ➢ metronidazole |

# 3.112.) GLAUCOMA

| Background | 95% of these are chronic, open angle |
|---|---|
| **Risk factors** | o family history<br>o African Americans |

---

**Chronic open-angle glaucoma**
- control intraocular pressure (IOP): medical or laser
- regular assessment of IOP and visual fields

---

**Acute angle-closure glaucoma (=medical emergency!)**

**1. Induce miosis**
- Pilocarpine or acetazolamide

**2. Reduce aqueous production**
- topical β-blocker or carbonic anhydrase inhibitor

**3. Laser iridotomy of <u>both</u> eyes**

## 3.113.) POSTSTREPTOCOCCAL GLOMERULONEPHRITIS

| | |
|---|---|
| **Background** | leading cause of acute nephritic syndrome |
| **Risk factors** | ○ streptococcal infection in children 2~6 years<br>(~15% risk after infection with nephritogenic strain) |
| **Prevention** | • treat streptococcal infections aggressively |
| **Management** | **1.** antihypertensives<br>**2.** salt restriction<br>**3.** diuretics<br><br>(Glucocorticoids are not useful) |

## 3.114.) GONORRHEA

| | |
|---|---|
| **Risk factors** | ○ multiple sexual partners |
| **Prevention** | • condoms<br>• identify and treat sexual partners |
| **Management** | ➢ single dose ceftriaxone<br>➢ plus 7-days doxycycline for chlamydia<br>• treat all partners |

# 3.115.) GOUT

| | |
|---|---|
| **Prevalence** | **Hyperuricemia:** 2~10% of population<br>**Gout:** 5% of patients with hyperuricemia |
| **Risk factors** | o obesity<br>o rapid cell turnover<br>➢ diuretics |

---

**1. Acute Gout**
- avoid aspirin!
- NSAIDs: indomethacin
- oral or intra-articular glucocorticoids
- colchicine only if NSAIDs and steroids contraindicated

**2. Chronic gout**
- reduce risk factors!
- allopurinol (inhibits uric aid synthesis)
- consider low-dose colchicine prophylaxis

 *Lifelong suppression of uric acid may be necessary if attacks recur.*

# 3.116.) GUILLAIN-BARRÉ SYNDROME

| | |
|---|---|
| **Risk factors** | ○ viral infection 1~3 weeks earlier |
| **Management** | 1. exclude cauda equina syndrome!<br>2. CSF is diagnostic<br>3. constant monitoring and support of vital functions<br>4. immune globulin infusion, plasmapheresis |
| **Prognosis** | • 30% require ventilatory assistance<br>• 10% have severe neurological residua<br>• 3% mortality |

# 3.117.) HEAT STROKE

| | |
|---|---|
| **Risk factors** | ○ elderly, bedridden patients<br>➢ use of anticholinergics, diuretics<br><br>○ salt and water deprivation<br>○ obesity<br>➢ alcohol |
| **Management** | 1. rapid cooling (ice water bath)<br>2. IV fluids and electrolytes |

 *Most patients recover within 30 minutes of collapse.*

# 3.118.) HEART FAILURE

**Sites of action for drugs used to treat heart failure:** Drugs that work in the heart enhance myocardial contractility, whereas drugs that work on other sites reduce either PRELOAD or AFTERLOAD.

Diuretics do so by decreasing blood volume. Vasodilators increase the space provided for the blood, thus reducing pressure.

Angiotensin converting enzyme (ACE) inhibitors block the synthesis of the vasoconstrictor angiotensin-II in the lungs. This also reduces aldosterone secretion from the adrenals, leading to water loss and reduction in blood volume.

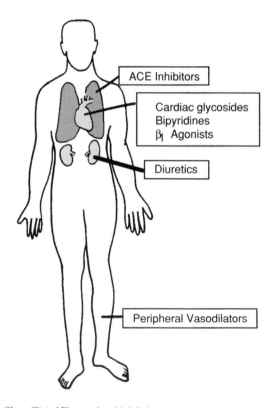

ACE Inhibitors

Cardiac glycosides
Bipyridines
β₁ Agonists

Diuretics

Peripheral Vasodilators

From Olson: *Clinical Pharmacology Made Ridiculously Simple*, MedMaster, 1994

## 1. Congestive heart failure

- Control excess salt and water:
  - sodium restriction
  - diuretics
- Vasodilators to reduce afterload:
  - ACE inhibitors
  - β-blockers or angiotensin-II receptor blockers.
- Improve cardiac contractility: digitalis

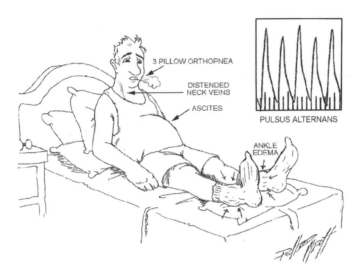

Modified from Chizner: *Clinical Cardiology Made Ridiculously Simple*, MedMaster, 2010

*Digitalis lessens symptoms, but has little effect on survival rate.*

# 3.119.) HEMOCHROMATOSIS

| Risk factors | o  male [1]<br>➤ alcohol (increases iron absorption) |
|---|---|
| 2° Prevention | • screen family members! |
| Management | **1.** low-iron diet<br>**2.** weekly phlebotomy to remove excess iron<br>(less frequent after iron stores normalize)<br>**3.** deferoxamine - iron chelation |

[1] *Clinical expression of disease is 10fold lower in women compared to men, due to protective effect of monthly menstruation.*

# 3.120.) HEMOPHILIA

| Background | hemophilia A is 10x more common than B |
|---|---|
| 2° Prevention | • genetic counseling |

---

**1. Factor concentrates**
- recombinant factor VIII (hem. A) or IX (hem. B)
- if not available, use heat-inactivated concentrate.
  (cryoprecipitate only as emergency backup)

**2. Other agents**
- DDAVP (vasopressin analogue, available as nasal spray)
  increases factor VIII levels by unknown mechanism

---

*10~20% of patients with hemophilia A will develop inhibitors (IgG) against factor VIII.*

# 3.121.) HEPATITIS

| | |
|---|---|
| **Prevalence**<br>(positive serology) | **HAV:** 20~40% (up to 100% in developing countries)<br>**HBV:** 5~10%<br>**HCV:** 1~2% |
| **Risk factors** | **HAV:** fecal-oral route, poor sanitation<br>**HBV:** body fluids, perinatal, male homosexuality<br>**HCV:** IV-drug abuse, blood transfusions |
| **Prevention** | **HAV:** good sanitation<br>**HBV:** screen all pregnant women<br>vaccinate infants at birth |
| **Management** | **1.** avoid hepatotoxins: alcohol, acetaminophen<br>**2.** no special treatment required in most cases<br>**3.** bed rest or dietary restrictions are unnecessary<br>**4.** HBV: lamivudine<br>**5.** HCV: interferon-α and ribavirin decrease risk<br>of chronic hepatitis |
| **Prognosis** | expect complete recovery in 3~6 months<br><br>**HBV:** 2% chronic active hepatitis → cirrhosis<br>5~10% asymptomatic HBsAg carriers<br><br>**HCV:** 50% chronic active hepatitis → cirrhosis |

*Risk of hepatitis C or HIV due to blood transfusion is negligible,*
*thanks to antibody and viral RNA testing of donor blood.*

## 3.122.) <u>HEPATOCELLULAR ADENOMA</u>

| | |
|---|---|
| **Background** | - exceedingly rare prior to oral-contraceptive era<br>- almost all occur in females |
| **Risk factors** | ➢ estrogen |
| **Management** | 1. discontinue oral contraceptives<br>2. avoid pregnancy (risk of rupture and bleeding)<br>3. if large → surgical removal |

## 3.123.) <u>HEPATOCELLULAR CARCINOMA</u>

| | |
|---|---|
| **Risk factors** | ○ males<br>○ liver cirrhosis (80% of cases)<br><br>○ HBV<br>○ HCV<br>➢ aflatoxin |
| **Prevention** | • HBV and HCV prevention<br>• consider AFP screening in high risk population |
| **Prognosis** | - radio- and chemotherapy usually unsuccessful<br>- liver transplantation limited by recurrence, metastases |

## 3.124.) <u>HEPATORENAL SYNDROME</u>

= renal failure in liver disease

| Risk factors | o  reduction in effective blood volume |
|---|---|
| **Prevention** | • avoid vigorous abdominal paracentesis<br>➢ avoid excessive diuresis<br>➢ albumin replacement |
| **Prognosis** | no effective therapy, almost always fatal |

## 3.125.) <u>HERPES SIMPLEX INFECTION</u>

| Prevalence | **HSV I:**  > 80% of population seropositive<br>**HSV II:**  20% of population seropositive |
|---|---|
| **Risk factors** | o  unprotected sexual intercourse<br>o  immune compromise (stress, illness)<br>o  neonates (via birth canal) |
| **Management** | **1.** avoid sexual contact while disease active<br>**2.** C. section if genital herpetic lesions present<br>**3.** acyclovir for serious or systemic disease |

*30% transmission rate if vaginal delivery during primary episode of mother.*

*HSV-II is an independent risk factor for transmission of HIV.*

# 3.126.) HERPES ZOSTER

Shingles

| Risk factors | ○ age<br>○ immunocompromise |
|---|---|
| Management | **1.** wet compresses to relief itching<br>**2.** analgesics, antihistamines<br>**3.** acyclovir for immunocompromised patients |

*Zoster patients may transmit Varicella virus to susceptible persons → chicken pox.*

# 3.127.) HIP FRACTURE

= fracture of proximal femur

| Risk factors | ○ osteoporosis |
|---|---|
| Prevention | • osteoporosis prophylaxis<br>• walking cane |
| Management | • internal fixation<br>• consider hip arthroplasty for femur neck fractures<br><br>• rapid mobilization is important! |

# 3.128.) HISTOPLASMOSIS

| | |
|---|---|
| **Risk factors** | **Bird droppings:**<br>○ excavation<br>○ bull dozing<br>○ cave exploration |
| **Management** | **1.** acute pulmonary disease: none required<br><br>**2.** chronic or disseminated disease : itraconazole<br>**3.** lifelong itraconazole maintenance for AIDS patients<br>**4.** amphotericin B for severe cases |
| **Prognosis** | **Pulmonary histoplasmosis:** resolves spontaneously<br>**AIDS patients:** up to 50% relapse despite therapy |

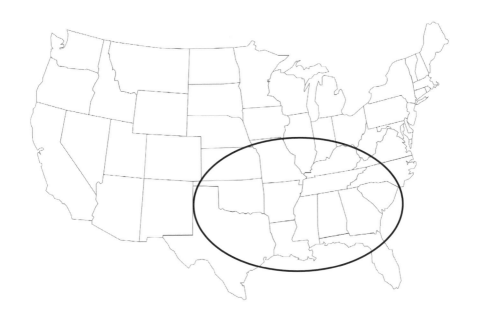

# 3.129.) <u>HIV INFECTION</u>

| | |
|---|---|
| **Background** | More than 30 million infected world wide<br>~50,000 new infections in US per year |
| **Risk factors** | **1. Sexual contact**<br>  o  homosexual<br>  o  heterosexual<br><br>**2. Percutaneous injury**<br>    needle stick<br><br>**3. Mucous membranes exposed to contaminated blood**<br><br>**4. Mother to infant** (vertical transmission)<br>  o  prenatal<br>  o  perinatal<br><br>**5. Breast feeding** |
| **Prevention** | • practice safe sex<br>• sexual counseling for teenagers<br>• needle exchange programs |
| **Prognosis** | life expectancy dramatically improved due to more aggressive drug regimens (=HAART) |

 *Risk of HIV infection after needle stick injury is about 1:250*

---

➤ Risk of HIV infection to fetus from HIV positive mother 10~40%.
➤ This can be reduced significantly if anti-HIV medication is given to the mother during pregnancy.

## 1. Initial evaluation

- HIV serology
- CD4 count
- assess presence of hepatitis, CMV, toxoplasma
- tuberculin test

- offer Pneumovax
- offer Hepatitis A and B vaccinations

## 2. Monitor development of disease

- CD4 count every 3-6 months
- or check viral RNA load

## 3. Antiretroviral therapy

- **start if CD4 < 500 or HIV RNA > 20,000**

**Reverse transcriptase inhibitors (nucleosides):**
- zidovudine (AZT)
- didanosine (ddI)

**Reverse transcriptase inhibitors (non-nucleosides):**
- nevirapine (NVP)

**Protease inhibitors:**
- saquinavir (SQV

## 4. If CD4 < 200

- trimethoprim-sulfamethoxazole prophylaxis for PCP

***HAART:*** *Always use combination therapy to prevent development of resistance. Initial therapy for example could be 2 or 3 nucleoside analogues plus a protease inhibitor.*

# 3.130.) HODGKIN LYMPHOMA

| Incidence | bimodal distribution: young adults + elderly |
|---|---|
| **Risk factors** | o male<br>o immunodeficiency<br>o (EBV infection in some cases) |

***B symptoms:*** *weight loss, fever, night sweats*

---

1. **Stage I (single lymph node region)**
2. **Stage II (several lymph node regions on same side of diaphragm)**
- if no B symptoms: radiate affected lymph node regions
- if B symptoms: chemotherapy plus/minus radiation
- consider adjuvant chemotherapy or hormonal therapy

---

3. **Stage III (several lymph node regions on both sides of diaphragm)**
4. **Stage IV (involves extranodal sites)**
- 6 to 8 cycles of chemotherapy:
**ABVD:** Adriamycin + Bleomycin + Vinblastine + Dacarbazine

---

5. **Relapse**
- consider high-dose chemotherapy / autologous stem cell transplant

 *Patients with splenectomy require Pneumovax vaccine.*

# 3.131.) HUNTINGTON'S CHOREA

| Risk factors | o family history |
|---|---|
| Management | • genetic counseling: ½ of offspring is potentially affected → offer DNA test to family members<br><br>➤ antidopaminergic drugs |
| Prognosis | • fatal within 20 years of onset<br>• early onset → more rapid progression |

# 3.132.) HYALINE MEMBRANE DISEASE

| Prevalence | 1~2% of newborns |
|---|---|
| Risk factors | o prematurity<br>o diabetic mother |
| Prevention | ➤ prenatal betamethasone accelerates lung maturation |
| Management | 1. exogenous surfactant<br>2. mechanical ventilation<br>(careful: avoid lung injury) |

# 3.133.) HYPEREMESIS GRAVIDARUM

| | |
|---|---|
| **Background** | some nausea and vomiting in ~75% of pregnancies |
| **Risk factors** | o  nulliparity<br>o  twin gestation<br>o  trophoblastic disease |
| **Management** | **1.** small frequent meals<br>**2.** avoid dehydration and nutritional depletion |
| **Prognosis** | •  increased risk of fetal anomalies and growth<br>•  risk of retardation if > 5% weight loss |

# 3.134.) ESSENTIAL HYPERTENSION

| | |
|---|---|
| **Prevalence** | 20% of population, of these 60% are salt-sensitive! |
| **Risk factors** | o  family history<br>o  obesity<br>➢  alcohol<br>➢  excess dietary sodium |

---

**1. If no other risk factors for coronary artery disease:**
- loose weight, exercise
- reduce $Na^+$ intake, increase $K^+$ intake

↓

**2. Pharmacotherapy**
- thiazide diuretic usually drug of choice
- β-blocker if angina or congestive heart failure

↓

**3. Pharmacotherapy**
- combine diuretic with any of the other class drugs

# 3.135.) HYPERTROPHIC CARDIOMYOPATHY

### Idiopathic Hypertrophic Subaortic Stenosis

| | |
|---|---|
| **Risk factors** | o family history in 50% of cases (often autosomal dominant) |
| **3° Prevention** | • avoid strenuous exercise<br>• avoid rapid standing<br>➢ avoid inotropic drugs<br>➢ avoid diuretics |

---

**1. Establish degree of abnormality**
- echocardiography → thickness of left ventricular wall
- treadmill exercise testing → ischemia? hypotension?
- consider ambulatory ECG → arrhythmias?

↓

**2. Pharmacotherapy**
- β-blocker or calcium channel blocker

↓

**3. Surgery**
- for patients with severe symptoms despite medication
- left ventricular myotomy: removal of part of the septum

*Hypertrophic cardiomyopathy is a common cause of sudden death in otherwise healthy young people and athletes.*

## 3.136.) IMPETIGO

usually *Staph. aureus*

| Background | preschool-age children (highly communicable!) |
|---|---|
| Risk factors | o tropical climate<br>o insect bites<br>o minor trauma |
| Prevention | • good hygiene |
| Management | **1.** topical antibiotic cream<br>**2.** oral erythromycin |

## 3.137.) ERECTILE IMPOTENCE

**1. distinguish psychological from organic causes**
• nocturnal penile tumescence

**2. Search for organic causes**
• peripheral vascular disease
• diabetic neuropathy
• endocrine
  - testicular failure
  - hyperprolactinemia

**3. Treatment options**
• Viagra (cGMP phosphodiesterase inhibitor)
• testosterone
• vacuum device to induce erection
• penile prothesis only if all others failed

# 3.138.) <u>INFECTIOUS ARTHRITIS</u>

| | |
|---|---|
| **Risk factors** | o *N. gonorrhea*: 70% of cases<br>o *Staphylococcus, Streptococcus, Haemophilus…*<br>o trauma<br>o joint prosthesis |
| **Prevention** | • STD prophylaxis |

# 3.139.) <u>INFERTILITY</u>

= failure to become pregnant after 1 year of unprotected intercourse

| | |
|---|---|
| **Prevalence** | 10~15% of all couples |
| **Risk factors** | male factors      ~ 40%<br>pelvic factors      ~ 30%<br>ovulation failure      ~ 20%<br>cervical factor      ~  5%<br>others      ~  5% |
| **Prevention** | • prevent STDs and pelvic inflammatory disease |
| **Management** | **1.** induce ovulation with clomiphene<br>**2.** artificial insemination<br>**3.** consider **in vitro fertilization** for:<br>  - tubal disease<br>  - oligospermia<br>  - sperm antibodies |

*Success rate of in vitro fertilization about 20~40% (age dependent).*
*Multiple gestation in ~30% of successful cases!*

# 3.140.) INFLUENZA

| | |
|---|---|
| **Background** | global epidemics (pandemics) every 10~15 years |
| | incubation period 1~5 days |
| | highest transmission rate at peak of symptoms |
| **Risk factors** | o crowded conditions, dormitories, prisons etc. |
| | o chronic heart/lung diseases predispose to complications |
| **Prevention** | **Seasonal influenza vaccine now recommended for all** |
| | Minimum age 6 month (or 2 years for live, attenuated vaccine) |
| **Management** | **1.** neuraminidase inhibitors effective only when given early |
| | **2.** symptomatic: fluids, antipyretics |
| **Complications** | bacterial pneumonia |

---

**Influenza A:**   Antigenic shift due to gene reassortment between animal and human viruses.

**Influenza B:**   Antigenic drift due to spontaneous mutations.

---

**H5N1** = "bird flu":    severe pneumonia, high fatality
**H1N1** = "swine flu":   highly transmittable, but often mild

# 3.141.) <u>INSOMNIA</u>

| | |
|---|---|
| **Prevalence** | 30% of adult population |
| **Risk factors** | o obesity<br>o chronic illnesses<br>➢ multiple drug use |
| **Management** | **SLEEP HYGIENE**<br>**1.** daily exercise<br>**2.** avoid caffeine<br>**3.** avoid late night snacks<br>**DRUGS**<br>**4.** if necessary, use short-acting hypnotics |

*Alcohol shortens sleep latency but hinders sleep maintenance (i.e. frequent awakening after sleep onset).*

# 3.142.) INTESTINAL OBSTRUCTION

| Risk factors | o previous abdominal surgery (75% of cases)<br>o external hernias<br>o inflammatory bowel disease |
|---|---|
| Management | • if peritoneal signs → emergency surgery |

 *Carcinoma is the most common cause of colonic obstruction.*


# 3.143.) INTUSSUSCEPTION

| Risk factors | o Henoch-Schönlein purpura<br>o leukemia, lymphoma<br>o cystic fibrosis<br>o recent upper respiratory infection |
|---|---|
| Management | • enema<br>• surgery if enema fails: prevent bowel infarction! |

 *Diagnosis: abdominal ultrasound. (Barium enema is both diagnostic and therapeutic, but carries a risk of bowel perforation! Careful!)*

# 3.144.) IRRITABLE BOWEL SYNDROME

| | |
|---|---|
| **Prevalence** | 10~20% of adult population<br>20~50% of adults with IBS seek medical attention |
| **Risk factors** | o  "learned illness behavior"? |
| **Management** | **Diarrhea-predominant**<br>➢ loperamide<br>**Constipation-predominant**<br>• high-fiber diet<br>• laxative: milk of magnesia<br><br>➢ consider herbal medicines<br>➢ consider low-dose antidepressant<br>➢ consider behavioral/relaxation therapy |
| **Prognosis** | lifelong condition, tends to lessen with age |

# 3.145.) ITP

**Immune-mediated destruction of platelets**

| | |
|---|---|
| **Risk factors** | **acute ITP:** children, female = male<br>**chronic ITP:** adults, female > male |
| **Management** | **1.** avoid platelet inhibitors (aspirin)<br>**2.** intravenous IgG<br>**3.** if platelets < 30,000 → glucocorticoids<br>**4.** if bleeding or < 10,000 → platelet transfusion<br>**5.** if medical therapy fails → splenectomy |

# 3.146.) JUVENILE IDIOPATHIC ARTHRITIS

| | |
|---|---|
| **Risk factors** | ○ HLA-B27, DR4, DR5, DR6 |
| **Management** | **1.** watch for uveitis → may lead to blindness<br>**2.** glucocorticoids:<br>   - inject joint if only one or two are involved<br>   - oral if systemic onset disease (Still's disease)<br>**3.** add methotrexate or sulfasalazine if steroids are<br>   not enough |
| **Prognosis** | up to 80% remission, variable mobility<br><br>Poorest prognosis if rheumatoid factor positive<br>and multiple joints affected. |

 *Most cases are rheumatoid factor negative.*

## 3.147.) KAPOSI SARCOMA
co-infection with human herpesvirus 8

| Background | 1981: in up to 50% of US AIDS patients was often the presenting sign today: much lower incidence |
|---|---|
| Risk factors | o HIV infection + male homosexuality o endemic Kaposi sarcoma in Africa |
| Management | • cryotherapy or electrocoagulation • treatment of Kaposi sarcoma does not prolong life in patients with HIV infection |

 *HIV-related Kaposi sarcoma: seen mostly in <u>homosexual</u> men.*

## 3.148.) KELOIDS

| Background | more common in black and Hispanic population |
|---|---|
| Risk factors | o family history o dark skin pigmentation o adolescence |
| Management | 1. local steroid injections 2. laser or cryotherapy |
| Prognosis | • high rate of recurrence • treatment often unsatisfying, leaving a flat and shiny scar |

# 3.149.) KIDNEY STONES

| Risk factors | o  high protein diet<br>o  low fluid intake<br>o  sedentary lifestyle<br>o  urinary tract infection<br><br>**hereditary:** cystinuria |
|---|---|
| Prevention | • increase fluid intake: urine output > 3L/day<br><br>• diet: reduce oxalate, calcium, purines and Vit. C |
| Management | ➤ Pain: NSAIDS, opiates<br><br>if <  4 mm    → may pass spontaneously<br>if < 20 mm    → lithotripsy<br>if > 20 mm    → surgery |

# 3.150.) LACTOSE INTOLERANCE

| Prevalence | American Indians:     100%<br>African Americans:     80%<br>Asians:                         80%<br>Caucasians:               < 10% |
|---|---|
| Management | **1.** avoid milk (yoghurt and cheese may be o.k.)<br>**2.** dietary lactase supplement<br>**3.** pre-hydrolyzed milk (LactAid) |

# 3.151.) LEAD POISONING

| | |
|---|---|
| **Background** | ~10% of preschool children have elevated blood lead levels! |
| **Risk factors** | o  pica<br>o  pre-1970 houses (leaded paint)<br>o  lead-soldered plumbing<br>o  industrial soil |
| **Management** | **1.** immediate chelation:    - EDTA<br>                                        - dimercaprol (BAL)<br><br>**2.** identify and eliminate source<br>**3.** report to OSHA if occupational |

# 3.152.) LEGIONNAIRES' DISEASE
*Legionella pneumophilia*

| | |
|---|---|
| **Risk factors** | o  smoking<br>o  alcohol abuse<br>o  chronic cardiopulmonary disease<br>o  immunosuppression |
| **Prevention** | •  avoid inhalation of aerosols<br>   (keep water heaters > 160° F) |
| **Management** | ➤  erythromycin, azithromycin |
| **Prognosis** | more severe than other "atypical pneumonias" |

# 3.153.) LEUKEMIA, ACUTE

| | |
|---|---|
| **Background** | most common type of cancer in children<br>**children: ALL** > AML<br>**adults:** **AML** > ALL |
| **Risk factors** | ➤ radiation exposure<br>➤ chemotherapy |
| **Prognosis** | **ALL in children:**   expect long term survival<br><br>**AML:**            60~80% remission rate<br>                  20~40% long term survival |

Treatment is complex and depends on type and subtype.
Here are examples of some "classic regimens":

---

**1. Induction (to achieve remission)**
- ALL: vincristine + prednisone + L-asparaginase
- AML: cytarabine + daunorubicin
- colony-stimulating factors to improve neutrophil count
- check bone marrow after 14 days

⬇

**2. Consolidation therapy (to eradicate residual blast cells)**
- same regimen as for induction, or single-agent high dose

⬇

**3. CNS prophylaxis (to prevent leukemic meningitis in ALL)**
- intrathecal methotrexate

⬇

**4. Maintenance therapy (to prevent relapse ALL)**
- mercaptopurine + methotrexate

---

 *AML: bone marrow transplant best hope for cure.*

# 3.154.) LEUKEMIA, CHRONIC

| Background | CLL is the most common form of leukemia overall |
|---|---|
| **Risk factors** | o age, male<br>o Philadelphia chromosome (t9:22) in CML |
| **Prognosis** | **CML:** often converts to AML within 2 years with poor prognosis<br><br>**CLL:** indolent for many years |

---

## CML

- **Imatinib** specifically inhibits tyrosinkinase activity of the bcr/abl oncogene
- assess molecular response: **bcr/abl/abl-ratio** by PCR is the "gold-standard"

- consider allogenic bone marrow transplant for patients > 50y.
- blast phase: treat like AML

---

## CLL

- **usually indolent:** early treatment does NOT improve survival
- chemotherapy if anemia or neutropenia or other signs of disease progression develop: - fludarabine
  - monoclonal antibodies

# 3.155.) <u>LISTERIOSIS</u>

| | |
|---|---|
| **Background** | • very high risk to fetuses and neonates<br>- miscarriage<br>- stillbirth<br>- potentially fatal infection after birth |
| **Risk factors** | o pregnancy, elderly, immunocompromised<br><br>**food:** soft cheese, pâté<br>uncooked hotdogs<br>undercooked chicken |
| **Prevention** | • avoid livestock during pregnancy<br>• avoid raw milk, soft chesses<br>• hotdogs, sliced deli meats |
| **Management** | ➢ ampicillin |

| | |
|---|---|
| **Pregnancy infection:** | mild disease in mother<br>high risk of fetal demise |
| **Neonatal infection:** | high risk of meningitis<br>high mortality |

238

# 3.156.) LIVER CIRRHOSIS

| | |
|---|---|
| **Risk factors** | o  alcohol<br>o  viral hepatitis B and C<br>o  genetic ($\alpha$1-antitrypsin deficiency, Wilson's etc.) |
| **Prevention** | •  limit alcohol<br>•  hepatitis B immunization<br>•  avoid needle sharing<br>•  practice safe sex |
| **Prognosis** | **Liver transplant:**<br>Failure          ~ 10%<br>Long-term survival   ~ 60% |

**1. Diet**
- normal caloric, normal protein diet
- reduce salt intake
- alcohol abstinence
- correct vitamin deficiencies

↓

**2. Ascites**
- diagnostic paracentesis: transudate
- reduce salt intake to ideally < 1g/day
- diuretics
- daily paracentesis
  (replace albumin IV)

↓

**3. Surgical options**
- consider TIPS: transjugular portosystemic stent
- consider liver transplant

# 3.157.) LUNG CANCER

#1 cause of cancer death in US, both men and women!

| Risk factors | o cigarette smoking<br>> 80% of lung cancer patients are smokers<br><br>o asbestos exposure |
| --- | --- |
| Prevention | • discontinue smoking<br>• large scale screening (chest X-ray) is NOT recommended |
| Prognosis | • 5-year mortality > 85% |

**1. Small cell carcinoma**
• radiation plus chemotherapy
• consider cranial radiation to prevent CNS metastasis

↓

**2. All other lung cancers**
• early stage → lobectomy
• late stage → radiation plus chemotherapy

↓

**3. Follow-up**
• Physical exam including chest X-ray every 3 months

# 3.158.) LYME DISEASE

most common vector-borne infection in US

| Risk factors | o tick infested areas<br>o summer months |
|---|---|
| Prevention | • protective clothing, repellent: DEET |
| Management | ➢ doxycycline |

 *Antibiotic prophylaxis (single-dose doxycycline within 72h) after tick bite in otherwise asymptomatic persons is controversial.*

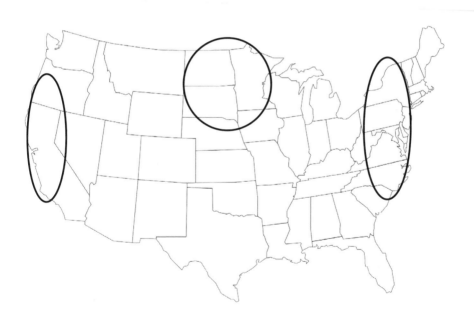

Disease is spreading and cases have been reported from most States.

# 3.159.) LYMPHOGRANULOMA VENEREUM

| Risk factors | o unprotected intercourse<br>o anal intercourse<br>o tropical countries |
|---|---|
| Management | ➢ doxycycline<br>• suggest HIV testing! |
| Prognosis | • may result in scarring, strictures and fistulas if not treated adequately |

# 3.160.) MAJOR DEPRESSIVE DISORDER

| Background | 15~20% of population have one episode during lifetime |
|---|---|
| Risk factors | o female<br>o family history<br><br>25% chance of mood disorder if one parent has bipolar type-1<br>70% chance of mood disorder if both parents have bipolar type-1 |
| Management | 1. Suicide risk? Does patient have specific plan?<br>2. serotonin reuptake inhibitors are first choice<br>   assess effectiveness after 4~6 weeks, taper slowly<br><br>3. if patient had several episodes → give maintenance medication<br>4. if patient is psychotic → add antipsychotic<br>5. consider psychotherapy |
| Prognosis | - 50% chance of recovery during first year<br>- better prognosis than bipolar disorder type-1 |

# 3.161.) MALARIA

| Risk factors | o transmitted by *Anopheles* mosquitos |
|---|---|
| Prophylaxis | ➤ chloroquine for travel to Central America<br>➤ mefloquine (or doxycycline) for all others |
| Management | **P. falciparum:**   mefloquine<br>**Others:**   chloroquine<br><br>**Prevention of relapse:** primaquine [1] |

[1] eradicates liver schizont of *P. vivax* and *P. ovale*

 *Mefloquine is effective in chloroquine resistant P. falciparum. It is safe during pregnancy.*

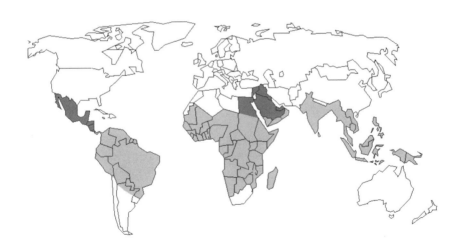

▮ Chloroquine sensitive    ▯ Chloroquine resistant *P. falciparum*

# 3.162.) MARFAN'S SYNDROME

| | |
|---|---|
| **Risk factors** | o  family history (autosomal dominant) |
| **Management** | **1.** regular echocardiography<br>**2.** β-blockers may delay aortic dilatation<br>**3.** antibiotic prophylaxis for endocarditis if heart murmurs or valve abnormalities are present |
| **Prognosis** | - aortic dissection & heart failure cause most of morbidity/mortality<br>- normal life span with appropriate surgical interventions |

# 3.163.) MASTALGIA

| | |
|---|---|
| **Background** | common in women with PMS |
| **Risk factors** | ➤ methylxanthines:<br>coffee, tea, chocolate |
| **Management** | • usually remits spontaneously<br>• for severe cases → consider low-dose tamoxifen [1] |
| **Prognosis** | • premenstrual mastalgia increases with age and generally subsides with menopause |

[1] *be aware of the slight increase in endometrial cancer rate with this drug!*

# 3.164.) MELANOMA

| | |
|---|---|
| **Risk factors** | o  fair skin complexion<br>o  history of blistering sunburns |
| **Prevention** | •  sunscreens, hats…!<br>(crucially important for <u>children</u> and <u>teenagers</u>!)<br>•  regular skin cancer checkups |
| **Management** | **1.** wide excision (margin based on tumor thickness)<br>**2.** consider lymph node resection<br>**3.** metastases: chemotherapy |
| **Prognosis** | **5-year survival**<br><br>**Stage I**  (<1mm thick)   ~ 90%<br>**Stage II**  (>1mm thick)  40 ~ 70%<br>**Stage III** (lymph nodes) 20 ~ 70%<br>**Stage IV** (metastases)   ~ 15% |

# 3.165.) MÉNIÈRE'S DISEASE

| | |
|---|---|
| **Risk factors** | o Caucasians<br>o stress<br>o allergy<br>o increased salt intake |
| **Management** | **1.** low-salt diet and diuretics<br>**2.** avoid ototoxic medications<br><br>**3.** 5% of patients may require surgery for incapacitating vertigo |
| **Prognosis** | • vertigo tends to improve with time<br>• hearing tends to decline with time<br>(loss of <u>low</u> frequencies) |

 *Don't overlook acoustic tumors, which may produce a clinically identical picture.*

# 3.166.) MENINGITIS

| | |
|---|---|
| **Risk factors** | **bacterial:** immunosuppression<br>head injury<br>alcoholism |
| **Management** | **empirical therapy:**<br>$3^{rd}$ generation cephalosporin + vancomycin<br>don't wait for results of CSF culture! |
| **Prognosis** | • bacterial is more severe than viral |

# 3.167.) MENTAL RETARDATION

| Definition | mild IQ < 70 |
|---|---|
| | moderate IQ < 50 |
| | severe IQ < 35 |
| | profound IQ < 20 |
| **Risk factors** | ~70% due to genetic abnormalities or congenital infections |
| | ~20% due to perinatal hypoxia, prematurity |
| | ~10% head trauma, CNS infections |
| **Management** | **mild:** basic job skills achievable |
| | **moderate:** group home living |
| | **severe:** needs supervision |
| | **profound:** needs extensive care |

 *A cause can be identified in 80% of severe cases but less than 50% of mild retardations.*


# 3.168.) MIGRAINE

| Risk factors | o family history, female > male |
|---|---|
| | o young age |
| **Prophylaxis** | ➤ β-blocker or topiramate if > 2 attacks/month |
| **Acute** | ➤ 5-HT agonists: sumatriptan |
| | ➤ ergot derivatives + caffeine (not for patients with peripheral vascular disease) |

# 3.169.) MITRAL STENOSIS
common in patients with rheumatic heart disease

| Risk factors | o  history of rheumatic fever |
|---|---|
| Management | **1.** rheumatic fever → bacterial endocarditis prophylaxis<br>**2.** consider balloon valvuloplasty in severe cases<br><br>**Atrial fibrillation**<br>**1.** β-blocker to slow heart rate<br>**2.** lifelong warfarin anticoagulation<br>    (to reduce risk of thrombus and stroke) |

# 3.170.) MITRAL VALVE PROLAPSE
most common cause of mitral regurgitation

| Risk factors | o  young females<br>o  cardiomyopathy |
|---|---|
| Management | **1.** if asymptomatic → observe<br>**2.** if palpitations → β-blockers<br>**3.** bacterial endocarditis prophylaxis if murmur<br>    is present or valve appears thickened on<br>    echocardiogram |

 *Endocarditis prophylaxis usually NOT necessary.*

# 3.171.) INFECTIOUS MONONUCLEOSIS
## Epstein-Barr virus infection

| | |
|---|---|
| **Prevalence** | 90~95% of adult population is seropositive |
| **Risk factors** | o higher socioeconomic groups [1]<br>o college students<br>o transmitted by saliva: kissing |
| **Management** | ➢ supportive care, NSAIDs<br>➢ avoid aspirin (Reye syndrome)<br>➢ avoid ampicillin (causes rash) |

[1] *larger probability of childhood infection in lower socioeconomic groups.*


# 3.172.) MGUS
## Monoclonal Gammopathy of Unknown Significance

| | |
|---|---|
| **Prevalence** | increasing with age<br>5% at age 70 years |
| **Management** | annual quantitative measurement of M-protein |
| **Prognosis** | 30% risk of multiple myeloma within 20 years ! |

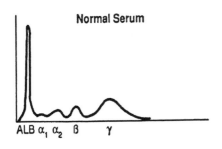 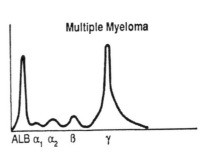

# 3.173.) MULTIPLE MYELOMA

| Risk factors | o age<br>o African Americans<br>o family history |
|---|---|
| Management | 1. if no symptoms ("smoldering"): observe<br>2. immunomodulatory<br>- lenalidomide + dexamethasone<br>3. consider high-dose chemotherapy with autologous stem cell transplantation<br>4. biphosphonate for patients with bone disease |

 *No CRAB = no treatment!*
*(calcium, renal failure, anemia, bone lesions)*


# 3.174.) MULTIPLE SCLEROSIS

| Risk factors | o Northern European descent<br>o living in temperate zone<br>o family history |
|---|---|
| Management | • avoid stress from hot weather<br><br>1. glucocorticoids for acute attack, taper carefully<br>2. interferon-β or glatiramer to slow progression<br>3. baclofen to reduce muscle spasms<br>4. anticholinergics to reduce voiding reflex |
| Prognosis | **better if:** early onset<br>relapsing-remitting course<br><br>**worse if:** action tremors present<br>primary progressive course |

# 3.175.) MUMPS

| | |
|---|---|
| **Risk factors** | o lack of immunization |
| **Prevention** | ➤ MMR vaccine at 15 months and 4~6 years<br>• virus is spread 2 days before until 10 days after parotitis |
| **Management** | • symptomatic only |
| **Prognosis** | • encephalitis in 1% of cases<br>• orchitis in 30% of postpubertal males (may decrease fertility, but sterility is rare) |

*MMR vaccine NOT recommended for pregnant women, patients receiving glucocorticoids or immunosuppressed (except HIV).*

## 3.176.) MUSCULAR DYSTROPHY

Duchenne is the most common form

| Risk factors | **Duchenne, Becker:** x-linked recessive<br>**myotonic dystrophy:** autosomal dominant |
|---|---|
| Prevention | **Duchenne, Becker:** determine maternal carrier status |
| Management | **1.** physical therapy, exercise<br>**2.** avoid obesity<br>**3.** prednisone slows decline in muscle strength<br>**4.** (gentamycin for a small subset of DMD patients) |

## 3.177.) MYASTHENIA GRAVIS

| Risk factors | ○ other autoimmune diseases |
|---|---|
| Management | **1.** acetylcholinesterase inhibitors: pyridostigmine<br>**2.** glucocorticoids<br>**3.** thymectomy |

*Thymus abnormalities (thymitis and thymoma) in 85% of patients. Since most improve with thymectomy, this procedure should be offered to all patients with myasthenia gravis.*

# 3.178.) <u>MYOCARDIAL INFARCTION</u>

**1. ECG / Labtests**
- ST elevation?
- Q inversion without ST elevation?

- cardiac troponin CTnT best marker for **acute infarction**
- creatinine kinase best marker for **reinfarction**

**2. Medications**
- **oxygen**
- **morphine**
- nitroglycerine to reduce pre- and afterload
- β-blocker to reduce $O_2$ demand

**3. Interventions**
- coronary angioplasty **within 90 mins**
- if not available: thrombolysis with tPA **within 6 hours**

**4. Post MI**
- Watch out for complications !!!
- Rehabilitation:
  - slowly progressive physical activity
  - aid patient to accept limitation
  - educate about risk factors of CHD

 *Aspirin has been shown to improve survival.*

# 3.179.) MI COMPLICATIONS

| | |
|---|---|
| **arrhythmia** | • dizziness, palpitations<br>• syncope |
| **congestive heart failure** | • dyspnea, orthopnea<br>• S3 gallop, S4 gallop<br>• rales, wheezes (cardiac asthma)<br>• cardiogenic shock |
| **myocardial rupture** | • tamponade, shock, death<br>• typically **occurs with small infarcts!** |
| **papillary muscle rupture** | • hyperacute onset pulmonary edema<br>• loud systolic murmur (mitral regurgitation) |
| **septal rupture** | • new onset holosystolic murmur |
| **ventricular aneurysm** | • reduced ejection fraction<br>• mural thrombi → arterial emboli |
| **pericarditis** | • **occurs 1~3 days after MI**<br>• pleuritic pain, non-responsive to nitrates<br>• diffuse ST elevations<br>• self-limited |
| **Dressler's syndrome** | • **occurs several weeks after MI**<br>• pericardial and pleural effusions<br>• fever, joint pain<br>• tends to recur |

# 3.180.) NARCOLEPSY

| Risk factors | o family history<br>o head trauma<br>o CNS infections |
|---|---|
| Management | 1. avoid long-distance driving<br>2. modafinil, methylphenidate or other amphetamine-like stimulant |

# 3.181.) NEURAL TUBE DEFECT

| Risk factors | o 1st trimester valproic acid<br>o folate deficiency<br>o family history of spina bifida |
|---|---|
| Prevention | ➢ folate supplementation during pregnancy |
| Management | ➢ involve neurosurgeon, urologist and orthopedic |
| Prognosis | ➢ normal IQ in > 80% open neural tube infants |

# 3.182.) NEUROBLASTOMA
most common extracranial solid tumor of childhood

| Risk factors | o genetic abnormalities<br>o fetal alcohol syndrome<br>➤ maternal phenytoin treatment |
|---|---|
| Management | 1. surgical excision<br>2. plus chemotherapy if advanced stage |
| Prognosis | **survival** 90% if age < 1 year<br>much less in children > 1 year |

# 3.183.) OBESITY

| Risk factors | o parental obesity<br>o pregnancy<br>o low socioeconomic status |
|---|---|
| Management | 1. life-style modification<br>2. exercise, low fat diet<br>3. surgery only for select, severely obese patients |
| Prognosis | long term maintenance of weight loss extremely difficult |

---

**BODY MASS INDEX:** weight (kg) / height$^2$ (m$^2$)

Overweight:      BMI >25 kg/m$^2$
Obese:      BMI >30 kg/m$^2$

# 3.184.) ONYCHOMYCOSIS

| Risk factors | o warmth<br>o moisture<br>o occlusive footwear |
|---|---|
| Prevention | • wear cotton socks<br>• avoid wool or synthetic fibers |
| Management | 1. establish diagnosis (culture, PAS stain)<br>2. topical or systemic antifungal (itraconazole)<br>3. nail can be removed surgically<br>   or dissolved with urea |
| Prognosis | over 50% relapse |

 *Over-the-counter antifungal creams are NOT effective.*


# 3.185.) OSGOOD SCHLATTER DISEASE

| Risk factors | o male<br>o rapid skeletal growth<br>o repetitive jumping sports |
|---|---|
| Management | • avoid sports that stress quadriceps muscle<br>  (basketball, bicycle riding) |
| Prognosis | resolves after skeletal maturation |

# 3.186.) OSTEOARTHRITIS

| Risk factors | o age<br>o obesity<br>o trauma<br>o (athletic activity ?) |
|---|---|
| Management | **1.** NSAID or selective COX-2 inhibitor: celecoxib [1]<br>**2.** intraarticular injection of glucocorticoid to reduce acute inflammation<br>**3.** weight loss if obese<br>**4.** exercise to strengthen muscles and maintain mobility |

[1] *Rofecoxib has been withdrawn from the market due to heart attack and stroke risk.*


# 3.187.) OSTEOMYELITIS

| Risk factors | o sickle cell disease<br>o IV drug use<br>o open fractures |
|---|---|
| Management | **1.** Antibiotic therapy (up to 1 year may be required):<br>**Acute osteomyelitis**<br>empirical antibiotic therapy against *Staph. aureus* (don't wait for results of culture)<br>**Chronic osteomyelitis**<br>identification of organism is crucially important<br><br>**2.** consider surgery to remove pus and necrotic tissue<br>**3.** avoid weight bearing until healed |

*Plain X-ray cheap but lower sensitivity.*
*Radionuclide scan has high sensitivity but expensive.*

# 3.188.) OSTEOPOROSIS

| | |
|---|---|
| **Prevalence** | up to 40% of elderly women<br>up to 10% of elderly men |
| **Risk factors** | o menopause<br>o inadequate dietary calcium/vit. D<br>o excessive dietary phosphate<br>o sedentary lifestyle<br><br>➤ glucocorticoids |
| **Management** | **1.** exercise<br>**2.** dietary calcium: 1500 mg/day<br>**3.** dietary Vit. D: 1000 IU/day<br>**4.** biphosphonate |

*Post-menopausal loss superimposed on age-related loss in females.*

# 3.189.) OTITIS MEDIA

| | |
|---|---|
| **Risk factors** | o day care setting<br>o exposure to cigarette smoke<br>o cleft palate |
| **Prevention** | • breast feeding<br>• eliminate smoking in household |
| **Management** | • often resolves spontaneously<br>➤ amoxicillin<br>➤ surgical drainage in severe cases |

*Otitis media is often painless and should be suspected in children who "don't pay attention".*

# 3.190.) OVARIAN CANCER

| | |
|---|---|
| **Risk factors** | o low parity<br>o late pregnancies<br>o family history<br>o Turner's syndrome |
| **Prevention** | ➢ pregnancy or oral contraceptives reduce risk by 30~60% |
| **Management** | **1.** staging<br>**2.** hysterectomy + bilateral salpingo-oophorectomy<br>**3.** chemotherapy: cisplatin + cyclophosphamide<br><br>CA125 test for recurrence, not for screening |

 *Overall high mortality (60%) due to late detection.*

# 3.191.) PANCREAS CANCER

| | |
|---|---|
| **Risk factors** | o smoking<br>o diabetes mellitus<br>o chronic pancreatitis<br>o African Americans |
| **Management** | **1.** if limited to head: pancreatomy or pancreaticoduodenectomy<br>**2.** plus chemotherapy and/or radiation<br>**3.** if inoperable: place stent to relief jaundice<br><br>**4.** opioids for pain! |

 *70% occur in the pancreas head.*

# 3.192.) PANCREATITIS

| | |
|---|---|
| **Risk factors** | o alcoholism<br>o cholelithiasis<br>o ERCP |
| **Prevention** | • avoid alcohol |
| **Management** | **ACUTE:**<br>**1.** NPO<br>**2.** admit patient to ICU<br>**3.** vigorous IV fluid<br>**4.** parenteral nutrition<br>**5.** prophylactic antibiotics<br>**6.** postpone cholecystectomy if possible<br><br>**CHRONIC:**<br><br>**1. exocrine** insufficiency: oral enzymes<br>**2. endocrine** insufficiency: may be deficient in both, insulin and glucagon<br>**3.** advocate alcohol abstinence |

**RANSON'S CRITERIA = Poor Prognosis**

**at admission:**
age > 55 years
WBC > 16,000/μL
glucose > 200 mg/dL
LDH > 400 IU/L
AST > 250 IU/L

**within 48hours:**
calcium < 8 mg/dL
hematocrit decreases > 10%
BUN increases > 5 mg/dL
albumin < 3.2 g/dL
$pO_2$ < 60 mmHg
fluid deficit > 4L

# 3.193.) PATENT DUCTUS ARTERIOSUS

| Risk factors | o prematurity<br>o high altitude<br>o maternal rubella |
|---|---|
| Management | **1.** indomethacin or aspirin accelerate closure<br>**2.** spontaneous closure after 3 months is rare<br>**3.** should be surgically closed before age of 3 years<br>if large or symptomatic |

 *Physiological closure should occur within 10~15h after birth.*

*Surgical closure recommended to prevent pulmonary hypertension and infectious endocarditis.*

# 3.194.) PELVIC INFLAMMATORY DISEASE

| Risk factors | o multiple sex partners<br>o use of IUD<br>o *C. trachomatis* and *N. gonorrhea* infection |
|---|---|
| Prevention | ➤ practice safe sex<br>➤ IUDs contraindicated if high risk sexual lifestyle |
| Management | **1.** get cervical culture<br>**2.** antibiotics |
| Prognosis | • chronic pain in 20%<br>• infertility in 15%<br>• 6fold higher risk of ectopic pregnancy |

# 3.195.) PEPTIC ULCER DISEASE

| | |
|---|---|
| **Background** | duodenal ulcer (DU) is clinically more common than gastric ulcer (GU) which often remains asymptomatic |
| **Risk factors** | o  cigarette smoking<br>➤  NSAIDs<br>➤  glucocorticoids<br><br>80% of patients with peptic ulcers harbor *H. pylori*<br><br>**No increased risk with:**<br>o  spicy food<br>o  alcohol, caffeine |
| **Management** | •  gastric ulcers should be biopsied to exclude gastric cancer<br><br>***H.Pylori* "Triple Therapy"**<br>**1.** proton pump inhibitor (PPI)<br>**2.** plus clarithromycin<br>**3.** plus amoxicillin (or metronidazole) |

*Most people (60% > 60 years) harbor H. pylori, but only some of them develop peptic ulcer disease.*

# 3.196.) PERNICIOUS ANEMIA

| | |
|---|---|
| **Risk factors** | o alcoholism<br>o lack of vit. B12 (strict vegetarian diet)<br>o gastrectomy<br>o fish tapeworm *D. latum*<br><br>o HLA-DR2 and HLA-DR4 |
| **Management** | ➤ lifelong parenteral Vit. B12 |
| **Prognosis** | early detection of anemia can prevent later neurological complications<br><br>**Anemia** is reversible with parenteral vit. B12<br>**Neurological effects** not reversible with vit. B12 |

# 3.197.) PERTUSSIS

| | |
|---|---|
| **Risk factors** | ○ lack of immunization |
| **Prevention** | ➢ DPT vaccine at 2,4,6 and 15 months and 6 years |
| **Management** | ➢ erythromycin |
| **Prognosis** | very serious in infants < 6 months |

*Prior to mass immunization, pertussis killed more children than measles, diphtheria, poliomyelitis and scarlet fever combined.*

# 3.198.) PHENYLKETONURIA

| | |
|---|---|
| **Risk factors** | ○ blond hair<br>○ blue eyes<br>○ fair skin |
| **Management** | **1.** routine neonatal screening (Guthrie test [1])<br>**2.** low-phenylalanine diet at least until age 12 years |
| **Prognosis** | • may lose up to 50 IQ points during first year of life if undiagnosed |

[1] *increasingly replaced by newer techniques such as mass spectroscopy*

## 3.199.) PHEOCHROMOCYTOMA
most are benign

| | |
|---|---|
| **Prevalence** | 0.1% of hypertensive patients |
| **Risk factors** | o MEN 2<br>o neurofibromatosis |
| **Management** | **1.** prior to surgery:<br>α-blocker: phenoxybenzamine<br>β-blocker: propanolol<br><br>**2.** surgical resection |


## 3.200.) PLACENTA PREVIA

| | |
|---|---|
| **Risk factors** | o prior placenta previa<br>o previous cesarean section<br>o previous induced abortions<br>o multiple gestation |
| **Management** | **1.** hospitalize if possible<br>**2.** have cross-matched blood ready<br>**3.** Cesarean delivery for all cases |

 *Perinatal mortality (15~20%) mainly due to prematurity.*

# 3.201.) PLAGUE

| Risk factors | o rats, fleas<br>o Western States of US |
|---|---|
| Prevention | • avoid contact with vectors<br>➤ post-exposure antibiotic for all contacts |
| Management | ➤ streptomycin or gentamicin |
| Prognosis | Plague pneumonia is fatal unless treated within hours |

Infection in a human occurs when a person is bitten by a flea that has been infected by biting a rodent that itself has been infected by the bite of a flea carrying *Yersinia pestis*. This way the disease is transmitted from wild rodents to domestic rodents to humans under conditions of crowding and poverty.

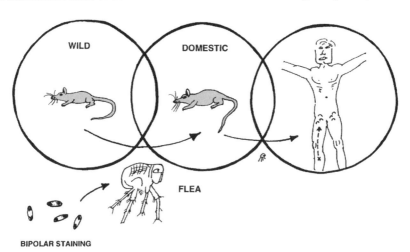

From Gladwin and Trattler: *Clinical Microbiology Made Ridiculously Simple*, MedMaster, 2008

 *All cases need to be reported to the CDC.*

# 3.202.) PNEUMONIA - BACTERIAL

| Risk factors | o viral infections<br>o hospitalization<br>o elderly<br>o COPD<br>o alcohol/smoking |
|---|---|
| Prevention | ➢ polyvalent pneumococcal vaccine<br>➢ annual influenza vaccine for everyone |
| Management | **Empirical antibiotics:**<br><br>➢ community acquired → clarithromycin[1] or doxycycline<br>➢ hospital acquired → broad spectrum cephalosporin or carbapenem[2].<br><br>➢ If *Staph. aureus* suspected: add vancomycin<br><br>*Switch to selective antibiotic once pathogen has been identified.*<br><br>[1] *macrolide*   [2] *β-lactamase resistant* |

# 3.203.) PNEUMONIA - MYCOPLASMA

| Risk factors | o army recruits<br>o college students<br>o other close communities |
|---|---|
| Management | ➢ macrolide or doxycycline |

# 3.204.) PNEUMONIA - PCP
*Pneumocystis Jirovecii*

| Prevalence | - most people have been exposed to PCP by age 3~4 years<br>- 50% of AIDS patients experience PCP pneumonia |
|---|---|
| Risk factors | o immunodeficiency |
| Prevention | ➢ CD4 < 200/mm$^3$: trimethoprim/sulfamethoxazole |
| Management | ➢ trimethoprim/sulfamethoxazole<br>➢ pentamidine if above is not tolerated |

*First episode mortality used to be as high as 50% but is decreasing due to improved awareness and therapy.*

# 3.205.) PNEUMONIA - VIRAL

90% of childhood pneumonias are viral (influenza, RSV and adenovirus). 30% of adult cases are viral, most are bacterial (pneumococcus).

| Risk factors | o immunocompromised<br>o close quarters |
|---|---|
| Prevention | • hand washing |
| Management | • mostly symptomatic<br>➢ never give aspirin to children or teenagers with fever (Reye syndrome) |

# 3.206.) POLIOMYELITIS

| | |
|---|---|
| **Background** | - last case in US was (imported) in 2005<br>- worldwide most cases due to live polio vaccine |
| **Prevention** | ➤ inactivated polio vaccine (Salk)<br>➤ live oral (Sabin) no longer used in US |
| **Management** | **1.** bed rest<br>**2.** physical therapy<br>**3.** intubation / tracheostomy may be needed |
| **Complications** | **meningitis**   in1% of cases<br>**paralysis**   in < 1% of cases |

*Many cases occur in contacts of persons who received the life oral poliovaccine (Sabin) which is used in developing countries due to low cost and effectiveness.*

# 3.207.) POLYCYSTIC KIDNEY DISEASE

| | | |
|---|---|---|
| **Genetics** | **adult form:**<br>**childhood form:** | autosomal dominant<br>autosomal recessive |
| **Associated with** | **adult form:**<br>**childhood form:** | intracranial aneurysms<br>hepatic fibrosis |
| **Management** | **1.** manage UTI and secondary renal hypertension<br>**2.** dialysis<br>**3.** kidney transplantation | |
| **Prognosis** | **adult form:** 50% end-stage renal disease at age 50<br>**childhood form:** renal failure at < 20 years of age | |


# 3.208.) POLYCYSTIC OVARY SYNDROME
### Stein-Leventhal Syndrome

| | |
|---|---|
| **Background** | common cause of oligomenorrhea / amenorrhea! |
| **Risk factors** | o obesity<br>o hypertension<br>o diabetes mellitus type 2 |
| **Management** | **1.** weight reduction and exercise to reduce insulin-resistance!<br>**2.** prevent endometrial and breast carcinoma by reducing estrogen levels:<br>- oral contraceptives<br>- progesterone to ensure regular shedding of the endometrium |

## 3.209.) POLYCYTHEMIA VERA

most common myeloproliferative disorder

| Risk factors | o Ashkenazi Jews<br>o elderly |
|---|---|
| Management | regular phlebotomy to reduce hematocrit to < 45% |
| Complications | acute leukemia in up to 2% of patients |

## 3.210.) POLYMYOSITIS / DERMATOMYOSITIS

| Risk factors | o female<br>o family history<br>o other autoimmune diseases |
|---|---|
| Management | 1. physical therapy<br>2. glucocorticoids<br>(taper carefully after patient improves)<br>3. if unresponsive → methotrexate |
| Prognosis | 50% full recovery<br>30% residual weakness<br>20% persistent active disease |

## 3.211.) PORPHYRIA
enzymatic defect of heme biosynthesis

| | |
|---|---|
| **Risk factors** | **Genetic**<br>**Attacks often triggered by:**<br>○ alcoholism<br>➤ oral contraceptives<br>➤ barbiturates<br>➤ carbamazepine<br>➤ sulfa drugs<br>➤ (many more) |
| **Prevention** | High-carbohydrate diet |
| **Management** | **1.** avoid precipitating drugs<br>**2.** avoid sunlight if photosensitive<br>**3.** acute attack: IV heme analogue |
| **Prognosis** | • acute intermittent porphyria up to 25% mortality<br>• other forms have excellent prognosis |

## 3.212.) POST-TRAUMATIC STRESS DISORDER

| | |
|---|---|
| **Risk factors** | ○ childhood neglect/abuse may predispose<br>○ war |
| **Prevention** | • crisis intervention immediately after trauma reduces incidence of later post-traumatic stress syndrome |
| **Prognosis** | • delayed onset → worse prognosis<br>• early treatment of acute phase → better prognosis |

# 3.213.) PROSTATE CANCER

| | |
|---|---|
| **Background** | most common malignancy in men<br>$2^{nd}$ most common cause of cancer death in men |
| **Risk factors** | o  hormonal<br>o  carcinogenic toxins<br>o  African Americans |
| **Prevention** | ➢ annual digital rectal exam for men > 50 years<br>➢ PSA screening |

*PSA elevated in 65% of cases.*
*PSA also elevated in BPH and prostatitis.*

---

**1. Stage 1 (non-palpable)**
**2. Stage 2 (palpable)**
- if patient's life expectancy is < 10 years and if the tumor is of low-grade, consider observation only
- radical prostatectomy, radiation
  (risk of impotence and urinary incontinence)

↓

**3. Stage 3 (extends through capsule)**
**4. Stage 4 (metastasis)**
- reduce androgens: GnRH agonist leuprolide
- chemotherapy

*Biphosphonate to reduce bone metastasis and pain.*

# 3.214.) PSEUDOMEMBRANOUS COLITIS

| | |
|---|---|
| **Risk factors** | ➢ Broad-spectrum antibiotics<br>o bowel surgery<br>o intestinal ischemia (shock etc.) |
| **Prevention** | ➢ keep course of antibiotics as brief as possible |
| **Management** | **1.** discontinue offending antibiotic<br>**2.** if symptoms persist: metronidazole or vancomycin |
| **Prognosis** | - often resolves spontaneously once wide-spectrum antibiotic is discontinued<br>- toxic megacolon has high mortality |

 ***The usual suspects:*** *clindamycin, ampicillin and cephalosporins.*

# 3.215.) PSITTACOSIS
*Chlamydia psittaci* infection

| | |
|---|---|
| **Risk factors** | o poultry plants, pet shop owners<br>(pet pigeons or parrots, chicken, turkeys....) |
| **Management** | ➢ prophylactic doxycycline if known exposure |

 *All birds are susceptible and may or may not be sick.*

# 3.216.) PSORIASIS

| | |
|---|---|
| **Risk factors** | ○ family history |
| | **Triggered by:**<br>○ local trauma/irritation<br>○ cold, stress<br>➢ glucocorticoid withdrawal |
| **2° Prevention** | • avoid trigger factors<br>➢ avoid antimalarial drugs |
| **Management** | ➢ topical fluorinated glucocorticoids<br>   (avoid systemic steroids → flare ups)<br><br>➢ UV-B or PUVA phototherapy<br>            (oral **P**soralen and **U**ltra**V**iolet-**A**)<br><br>➢ Tar shampoos |

# 3.217.) PUERPERAL INFECTION

| | |
|---|---|
| **Risk factors** | ○ premature rupture of membranes<br>○ prolonged labor<br>○ Cesarean section<br>○ urinary tract infections |
| **Prevention** | • good prenatal care<br>• patient education regarding rupture of membranes<br>➢ antibiotic prophylaxis for C. section if at high risk |
| **Management** | ➢ broad spectrum antibiotics<br><br>**If fever does not subside, consider:**<br>- retained products of conception<br>- abscess<br>- septic pelvic thrombophlebitis |

# 3.218.) PULMONIC VALVE STENOSIS

| | |
|---|---|
| **Risk factors** | ○ family history<br>○ other congenital heart defects |
| **Management** | • balloon valvuloplasty only if symptomatic |

# 3.219.) PYELONEPHRITIS

| | |
|---|---|
| **Background** | 80% of cases are hospital acquired |
| **Risk factors** | o indwelling catheter<br>o nephrolithiasis<br>o diabetes mellitus |
| **Prevention** | ➢ encourage fluid intake |
| **Management** | **Empirical antibiotics against _Enterobacteriaceae_**<br><br>**mild disease:**<br>- oral fluoroquinolones drug of choice<br>- trimethoprim/sulfamethoxazole alternative<br><br>**severe disease:**<br>1. urine and blood culture<br>2. antibiotics<br>- 3$^{rd}$ generation cephalosporins<br>- aminoglycosides<br>- fluoroquinolones<br><br>➢ imaging only if not responding to antibiotics |

 *10~15% of patients with indwelling catheters develop bacteriuria.*

# 3.220.) PYLORIC STENOSIS

| Risk factors | o Caucasians<br>o first born<br>o male |
|---|---|
| Management | • myotomy is effective in > 99% |

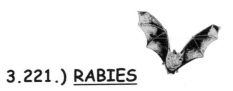

# 3.221.) RABIES

| Risk factors | **US:**       bats, skunks, raccoons<br>**outside of US:** dogs |
|---|---|
| Management | **Post-exposure:**<br>**1.** local wound cleansing<br>**2.** passive immunization on day 1<br>**3.** active immunization on days 1, 3, 7, 14 and 28 |

*Confine animal for 10 days. If it remains healthy, rabies is very unlikely.*

# 3.222.) RAYNAUD'S PHENOMENON

| Risk factors | o female<br>o smoking<br>o autoimmune connective tissue diseases |
|---|---|
| Management | 1. avoid trauma to fingertips<br>2. avoid exposure to cold<br>3. stop smoking |

*Raynaud's phenomenon is often the presenting symptom of scleroderma.*

# 3.223.) REITER'S SYNDROME

| Risk factors | o HLA-B27<br>o non-gonococcal urethritis<br>o bacterial dysenteriae |
|---|---|
| Management | 1. treat *Chlamydia* infection with tetracycline<br>2. NSAIDs for arthritis<br>3. physical therapy |

# 3.224.) RENAL CELL CARCINOMA

| | |
|---|---|
| **Risk factors** | o cadmium<br>o asbestos<br>o smoking<br>o obesity |
| **Management** | • radical nephrectomy<br>(kidney + adrenal gland + lymph nodes)<br><br>➤ immunotherapy: tyrosine kinase inhibitors<br>➤ chemotherapy not very effective |
| **Prognosis** | **5-year survival**<br><br>**Stage I** (confined to kidney)       - 90%<br>**Stage II** (extends through capsule)   - 50%<br>**Stage III** (involves hilar lymph nodes) - 20%<br>**Stage IV** (invades adjacent organs)   -  5% |

# 3.225.) RETINAL DETACHMENT

| Risk factors | o myopia<br>o trauma<br>o retinal degeneration |
|---|---|
| Management | 1. ophthalmic emergency<br>2. regular ophthalmologic exam if at high risk<br>3. seal retinal holes with laser |

 *Watch out for flashes or visual field abnormalities in patients with severe myopia!*

# 3.226.) RETROLENTAL FIBROPLASIA
leading cause of childhood blindness in US

| Risk factors | o low birth weight<br>o prematurity<br>o supplemental oxygen |
|---|---|
| Prevention | • reduce risk factors a/w low birth weight: smoking, alcohol, drug abuse...<br>➢ be careful with oxygen therapy<br>➢ vitamin E (anti-oxidant) |
| Management | • may need laser coagulation to prevent retina detachment |

# 3.227.) REYE'S SYNDROME
= fatty liver plus encephalopathy

| Risk factors | o  Influenza B<br>o  viral infections<br>➢ **aspirin, salicylates in children and teens** |
|---|---|
| Management | **1.** supportive<br>**2.** mannitol to reduce cerebral edema |

# 3.228.) RHEUMATOID ARTHRITIS

| Risk factors | o  female<br>o  Native Americans<br>o  HLA-DR4 |
|---|---|
| Management | **Anti-inflammatory**<br>➢ NSAIDs<br>➢ glucocorticoids<br><br>**Disease-modifying drugs**<br>➢ methotrexate (low-dose)<br>➢ sulfasalazine<br>➢ rituximab<br>   (monoclonal antibody against B cells)<br>➢ TNF inhibitors |

*Disease-modifying drugs should be given early to slow the irreversible joint destruction! Don't expect beneficial effects until 2~6 months after initiating therapy.*

# 3.229.) ROSEOLA
### Exanthema Subitum = 6th disease

| | |
|---|---|
| **Prevalence** | 75% of children are seropositive for HHV-6 by age 1. |
| **Background** | • rash appears after becoming afebrile<br>• once afebrile no longer infectious |

# 3.230.) RUBELLA
### German Measles

| | |
|---|---|
| **Background** | Most US cases "imported" from Latin-/South America.<br>10~30% of young adults are susceptible in US! |
| **Risk factors** | o inadequate immunization |
| **Prevention** | ➤ MMR vaccine at 15 months and 4~6 years<br>(persons who receive vaccine do not transmit virus) |
| **Complications** | **Congenital Rubella Syndrome**<br>Severe congenital diseases (heart defects, cataract, glaucoma) occur if maternal infection happens during first trimester of pregnancy. |

---

**Pregnant women exposed during first trimester:**
1. If seropositive: immunity is present → little risk.
2. If seronegative: get second test in 4~6 weeks.
   If test converts: consider therapeutic abortion.

---

# 3.231.) RUBEOLA
### Measles

Was declared eliminated in USA in 2000.

| | |
|---|---|
| **Risk factors** | o inadequate immunization (Americas) |
| **Prevention** | ➤ MMR vaccine at 15 months and 4~6 years |
| **Management** | • isolate for 1 week after rash onset<br>• bed rest until afebrile<br>• fluids<br>➤ antipyretics |
| **Complications** | **Encephalitis:** 1:1,000, 10% mortality<br>**SSPE:** extremely rare, 5~15 years after infection |

# 3.232.) SARCOIDOSIS

| | |
|---|---|
| **Risk factors** | o African Americans<br>(10 fold higher risk than Caucasians) |
| **Management** | • observe<br>➤ severe pulmonary dysfunction → glucocorticoids |
| **Prognosis** | - spontaneous resolution in 80%<br>- active/recurrent disease in 20% |

# 3.233.) SCARLET FEVER

| Prevention | ➤ prophylactic penicillin after exposure NOT recommended<br>➤ treat group-A β-hemolytic streptococcal pharyngitis<br>(mostly to prevent complications) |
|---|---|
| Management | ➤ penicillin<br>• children should not return to school until after 24h<br>of treatment |

# 3.234.) SCHIZOPHRENIA

| Incidence | 1% of population at some point of their life |
|---|---|
| Risk factors | ○ monozygotic twin concordance     - 40%<br>○ dizygotic twin concordance      - 10%<br>○ low socioeconomic status<br>○ severe stress often serves as a trigger |
| Management | **1. Neuroleptics (act on D-2 receptors)**<br>- Chlorpromazine: low-potency antipsychotic<br>- Haloperidol: high-potency antipsychotic<br>- Clozapine: fewer extrapyramidal side effects<br>           risk of agranulocytosis: monitor WBC<br>**2. Maintenance**<br>- for 1~2 years after first episode<br>- IM depot haloperidol or fluphenazine<br><br>**3.** Enroll patient in a community-based support program |

 ***Dyskinesias:*** *Acute dystonia (within hours of treatment) and Parkinsonism (weeks to months of treatment) are usually reversible.*

 *Tardive dyskinesia (occurring after many months) is irreversible.*

# 3.235.) SEBORRHOIC DERMATITIS

| | |
|---|---|
| **Risk factors** | ○ genetic predisposition<br>○ emotional stress triggers flare-ups |
| **Management** | **1.** ketoconazole cream<br>**2.** daily selenium sulfide shampoos |
| **Prognosis** | **Infants:** resolves after 6~8 months<br>**Adults:** chronic, lifelong |

# 3.236.) SEPSIS

| | |
|---|---|
| **Risk factors** | ○ age<br>○ indwelling catheters |
| **Prevention** | ➤ pneumococcal vaccine for elderly<br>• hand washing by hospital personnel<br>• catheter care |
| **Management** | **1.** stabilize: airways, breathing, circulation<br>**2.** get blood cultures before antibiotics<br>(aerobic and anaerobic)<br>**3.** empiric antibiotics against:<br>- *Staph. aureus*<br>- *E.coli*<br>- *Pseudomonas aeruginosa* |

# 3.237.) SIALOADENITIS

| Risk factors | o dehydration<br>o hypercalcemia |
|---|---|
| Management | 1. hydration<br>2. suck on candy<br>3. antistaphylococcal antibiotics |

# 3.238.) SICKLE CELL DISEASE

| Prevalence | 1 : 500 African Americans have disease<br>1 : 12 African Americans have trait<br>(= heterozygous carriers) |
|---|---|
| Risk factors | **vaso-occlusive crisis**<br>o dehydration<br>o hypoxia<br>**aplastic crisis**<br>o severe infections<br>o folic acid deficiency<br>**hemolytic crisis**<br>o bacterial infections<br>o exposure to oxidant drugs |

**Prevent infections and complications**
- penicillin prophylaxis for children
- pneumococcal vaccination
- hydroxurea: increases HbF, decreases HbS polymers
- bone pain plus fever → suspect osteomyelitis
- remove spleen if repeated infarction occurs

**Anemic crisis**
- bed rest, oxygen
- consider blood transfusion

# 3.239.) SILICOSIS

| Risk factors | o metal mining<br>o pottery making<br>o sandstone cutting |
|---|---|
| Prevention | • avoid dust exposure<br>• substitutes for silica |
| Complications | increased risk for tuberculosis |

*The classic "eggshell" pattern (calcification of hilar nodes) takes 10~20 years to develop.*


# 3.240.) SLEEP APNEA

| Prevalence | 5% of population |
|---|---|
| Risk factors | o obesity<br>o nasal obstruction<br>o macroglossia |
| Management | • weight loss<br>• avoid alcohol and sedatives<br>➤ CPAP: continuous positive airway pressure at night<br>➤ for severe cases: remove tonsils, adenoid, uvula |

*Obstructive sleep apnea is much more common than central sleep apnea.*

*Suspect in every patient with history of snoring and excessive daytime sleepiness.*

# 3.241.) SQUAMOUS CELL CARCINOMA

| | |
|---|---|
| **Risk factors** | o sun exposure<br>o fair skin |
| **Prevention** | • sunscreens, hat... |
| **Management** | • excision (Mohs micrographic surgery) |
| **Prognosis** | 1~2% metastatic potential<br>- higher if on ears or lips<br>- lower if arising within actinic keratosis [1] |

[1] *Actinic keratosis: cryosurgery + sun protection to prevent progression*

# 3.242.) STASIS DERMATITIS/ULCER

| | |
|---|---|
| **Risk factors** | o deep vein thrombosis<br>o previous pregnancy<br>o trauma<br>o obesity |
| **Management** | 1. elevate ankle<br>2. compression stockings to prevent edema<br>3. topical lubricant<br>4. stasis ulcer: zinc oxide paste |

# 3.243.) STROKE

| | |
|---|---|
| **Background** | 90% of cases due to ischemia-infarction<br>10% of cases due to hemorrhage |
| **Risk factors** | o age<br>o hypertension<br>o smoking<br>o diabetes<br>o antiphospholipid antibodies |
| **Prevention** | • stop smoking<br>• control blood pressure and diabetes<br>• exercise |

 *All stroke patients should be treated in <u>stroke unit</u>!*

---

**1. Acute stroke**
- get CT to exclude intracranial hemorrhage
- plasminogen activator for all patients within 3h of onset – unless contraindicated!
- low-dose aspirin improves outcome

**2. Supportive care**
- normalize blood pressure
- provide adequate nutrition
- watch for dehydration
- prevent deep vein thrombosis (heparin, mobilization)

**3. Rehabilitation**
- start early, within the first few days!

---

 *Heparin and warfarin increase risk of intracranial hemorrhage.*

# 3.244.) SUBARACHNOID HEMORRHAGE

| | |
|---|---|
| **Risk factors** | o saccular aneurysm<br>o polycystic kidney disease (adult type)<br>o AV malformation<br>o hypertension |
| **Prevention** | • prophylactic surgery of incidental aneurysms |
| **Management** | **1.** bed rest<br>**2.** lower blood pressure<br>**3.** phenytoin to prevent seizures<br>**4.** aneurysms tend to rebleed → early surgery |

*Up to 3% of the population harbor saccular aneurysms (based on autopsy studies).*


# 3.245.) SUBDURAL/EPIDURAL HEMORRHAGE

| | |
|---|---|
| **Risk factors** | o motor vehicle accidents<br>o falls<br>o alcoholism<br>o epilepsy |
| **Prevention** | • trauma prevention<br>➢ avoid alcohol |
| **Management** | **1.** if minor: glucocorticoids, observe<br>**2.** otherwise surgical evacuation |

*Subdural hemorrhage can occur without direct trauma (for example whiplash injuries).*

# 3.246.) SUDDEN INFANT DEATH SYNDROME

| | |
|---|---|
| **Risk factors** | o  Minority groups<br>o  low socioeconomic status<br>o  **prone sleeping position** |
| **Prevention** | •  "back to sleep"<br>healthy infants should sleep on their back! |
| **Management** | •  parents suffer from grief and feelings of guilt:<br>provide supportive psychological counseling |
| **Prognosis** | siblings have a 2~3fold higher risk |

 *A cause of death can be identified by autopsy in only 20% of cases.*

# 3.247.) SUICIDE

| | |
|---|---|
| **Background** | - 2$^{nd}$ leading cause of death in adolescents<br>- highest incidence in elderly > 65 years<br>- 80% of victims have seen physician in past 6 months |
| **Risk factors** | o depression<br>o psychotic disorders<br>o alcoholism<br>o drug abuse<br>o previous attempts |
| **Management** | **1.** hospitalize<br>**2.** if overdose: remove drugs, prevent absorption, antidotes<br><br>**3.** get psychiatric evaluation |
| **Prognosis** | 10% of all attempts are "successful" |

 *Homicide is the leading cause of death in black male adolescents.*

## SOME ANTIDOTES:

| INTOXICATION | ANTIDOTE |
|---|---|
| acetaminophen | N-acetylcysteine |
| opiates | naloxone |
| benzodiazepines | flumazenil |
| methanol, ethylene glycol | ethanol |
| CO | 100% O$_2$ |
| cyanide | amyl nitrate |
| lead | EDTA |
| warfarin | fresh frozen plasma, vitamin K |
| heparin | protamine sulfate |
| organophosphates | pralidoxime, atropine |
| atropine | physostigmine |

# 3.248.) SYPHILIS

| Risk factors | o multiple sex partners<br>o IV drug abuse<br>o male homosexuality |
|---|---|
| Prevention | • practice safe sex |
| Management | ➢ penicillin<br>• no sex for 7~10 days<br>• report to health agency |

*Jarisch-Herxheimer reaction (fever, myalgia, headache) in 50% of patients within 2h of treatment.*


# 3.249.) SYSTEMIC LUPUS ERYTHEMATOSUS

| Risk factors | o African Americans, Asians, Hispanics<br>o HLA-DR2, DR3, DQ3 |
|---|---|
| Management | **SKIN**<br>• avoid sun if photosensitive<br>➢ malar rash: hydroxychloroquine<br><br>**ARTHRITIS, SEROSITIS**<br>➢ try NSAIDs first<br>➢ short course of glucocorticoids<br><br>**KIDNEYS**<br>• renal biopsy to determine therapy and prognosis<br>➢ high dose glucocorticoids |

*Drugs known to induce SLE are NOT contraindicated in patients with idiopathic SLE.*

# 3.250.) TEMPORAL ARTERITIS

| Risk factors | o age<br>o polymyalgia rheumatica |
|---|---|
| **Management** | • if suspicion: treat first - biopsy second<br><br>➤ high-dose glucocorticoid for 1 month<br>  taper carefully when ESR declines |
| **Prognosis** | • high risk of blindness and stroke if untreated |

# 3.251.) TEMPOROMANDIBULAR JOINT SYNDROME

| Risk factors | o chronic teeth grinding<br>o dental malocclusion<br>o stress |
|---|---|
| **Management** | **1.** tension relief<br>**2.** orthodontics |

# 3.252.) TESTICULAR CANCER

| | |
|---|---|
| **Risk factors** | o age 20~40 years<br>o Caucasians<br>o history of cryptorchidism<br>o higher socioeconomic status<br>o unmarried |
| **Management** | **SEMINOMAS**<br>➤ orchiectomy plus radiotherapy<br>➤ chemotherapy for advanced stages<br><br>**NON-SEMINOMAS**<br>➤ orchiectomy plus chemotherapy |
| **Prognosis** | - infertility<br>- 70~90% cure, even in advanced cases |

 *Consider cryopreservation (sperm-bank) prior to treatment.*


# 3.253.) TESTICULAR TORSION

| | |
|---|---|
| **Risk factors** | o adolescence<br>o winter season |
| **Management** | **1.** distinguish from inflammation (Doppler ultrasound)<br>**2.** immediate surgery |
| **Prognosis** | • < 85% testicular salvage if duration > 6 hours<br>• 2/3 of salvaged testicles will atrophy later |

 *Any child/adolescent with scrotal pain should be assumed to have torsion unless proven otherwise.*

# 3.254.) TETANUS

| | |
|---|---|
| **Risk factors** | o burns<br>o frost bite<br>o skin ulcers<br>o drug addiction |
| **Prevention** | ➤ maintain active immunization<br>(toxoid every 10 years) |
| **Management** | **1.** give tetanus immune globulin IM immediately<br>**2.** penicillin for clostridial infection<br>**3.** diazepam to reduce spasms<br>**4.** active immunization after patient recovers |

Signs of Tetanus:

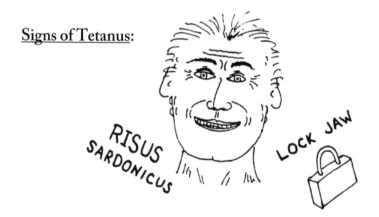

From Gladwin and Trattler: *Clinical Microbiology Made Ridiculously Simple*, MedMaster, 2008

# 3.255.) THALASSEMIA

| | |
|---|---|
| **Risk factors** | o Mediterranean<br>o Middle East<br>o Southeast Asia |
| **Management** | **mild:**    no treatment necessary<br>**HbH:**    folate supplementation<br>**severe:**  regular blood transfusions<br>            folate supplementation<br>            iron chelation<br><br>Hypersplenism may require splenectomy |
| **Prognosis** | **Thalassemia minor:**  normal life expectancy<br>**Thalassemia major:**  life expectancy < 20 years |

 *Hemoglobinopathies are extremely heterogeneous on the molecular level (over 600 known mutations).*

# 3.256.) THROMBOPHLEBITIS

| | |
|---|---|
| **Risk factors** | o immobilization<br>o IV catheters (especially lower extremities)<br>o IV drug abuse |
| **Prevention** | • replace IV cannulas every 48~72 hours |
| **Management** | • warm compresses<br>➢ NSAIDs<br><br>➢ anticoagulants usually not needed<br>➢ antibiotics not needed either (unless septic abscess) |

# 3.257.) THYROID CANCER

| Incidence | papillary > follicular > anaplastic |
|---|---|
| **Risk factors** | **papillary carcinoma:**   head and neck irradiation<br>**medullary carcinoma:**  MEN 2 |
| **Management** | **1.** thyroidectomy<br>    - protect parathyroids!<br>    - watch out for recurrent laryngeal nerves!<br>**2.** radioactive iodine to destroy thyroid remnants<br>**3.** give thyroid hormone to suppress TSH<br>**4.** for anaplastic cancer → add radiation therapy |
| **Prognosis** | papillary (best) > follicular > anaplastic |

# 3.258.) TOURETTE'S SYNDROME
### motor and vocal tics

| Risk factors | o  male<br>o  family history (up to 30% have motor ticks) |
|---|---|
| **Management** | ➢  α2-agonist (clonidine) to suppress tics |
| **Prognosis** | 50% improve spontaneously during adolescence |

 *Intelligence does not deteriorate!*

# 3.259.) TOXIC SHOCK SYNDROME
Staph. aureus

| Risk factors | o young women<br>o tampons<br>o nasal packing |
|---|---|
| Prevention | • frequent tampon change |
| Management | **1.** treat shock<br>**2.** vancomycin [1] + clindamycin IV<br><br>**3.** surgical intervention for TSS due to necrotizing fasciitis ("flesh eating bacteria") [2] |

[1] *because of emergence of methicillin-resistant Staph. aureus (MRSA)*
[2] *Streptococcus pyogenes causes a toxic shock-like syndrome*
*(= TSS + severe soft tissue necrosis)*


# 3.260.) TOXOPLASMOSIS

| Risk factors | **Transplacental transmission:**<br>**1st trimester:** lowest transmission rate (15%)<br>severe neonatal disease<br>**3rd trimester:** highest transmission rate (65%)<br>asymptomatic neonates |
|---|---|
| Prevention | • avoid cat feces<br>• avoid raw meat, raw eggs |
| Management | ➢ pyrimethamine plus sulfadiazine |
| Prognosis | - acute toxoplasmosis is usually asymptomatic<br>- high risk of encephalitis in AIDS patients |

*Women who are seropositive before pregnancy are protected against acute infection (i.e. no risk of congenital disease for fetus).*

# 3.261.) TRICHINOSIS

| Risk factors | <ul><li>undercooked pork or game</li><li>cooking at 71°C for 1 min. kills *Trichinella* larvae</li></ul> |
|---|---|
| Management | <ul><li>self-limited disease</li><li>➢ NSAIDs for muscle pain</li></ul> |
| Prognosis | <ul><li>most infections asymptomatic</li><li>rarely enteritis or myositis</li></ul> |

# 3.262.) TRICHOMONIASIS

| Risk factors | <ul><li>multiple sex partners</li></ul> |
|---|---|
| Prevention | <ul><li>practice safe sex</li><li>treat partners</li></ul> |
| Management | <ul><li>➢ metronidazole</li></ul> |

 *Most men are asymptomatic.*

# 3.263.) TRISOMY 21

Down syndrome

| | |
|---|---|
| **Risk factors** | **Maternal Age:**<br>1:2000   at age 20<br>1:200    at age 35<br>1:20     at age 45 |
| **Prevention** | **Triple screen test** for all pregnant women:<br>- AFP<br>- hCG<br>- estriol<br><br>**Amniocentesis** at 13~15 weeks if high risk |
| **Prognosis** | • 1% recurrence risk<br>  (much higher if due to translocation)<br><br>• premature aging<br>• clinical Alzheimer's disease after age 35 in<br>  30% of Down patients |

*Risk of fetal loss with amniocentesis is < 0.1%*
*Risk of fetal loss with chorionic villus sampling is ~1%*

# 3.264.) <u>TUBERCULOSIS</u>

Most infected people never develop active tuberculosis. However, multi drug-resistance is increasingly common and TB remains a major health threat worldwide.

| | |
|---|---|
| **Risk factors** | o  urban, homeless, close contact with infected<br>o  immunosuppression |
| **Prevention** | •  annual PPD skin test for high risk persons<br>➤  BCG vaccine has inconsistent efficacy |

---

**1. Diagnosis**
- Chest X-ray
- Get several sputums for culture and sensitivity testing
- Notify local health department

↓

**2. Latent tuberculosis**
- **Goal:** prevent active TB in those already infected
- **Isoniazid prophylaxis if:**
  PPD > 15 mm in low risk persons
  PPD > 10 mm in high risk persons
  PPD >  5 mm in HIV patients

↓

**3. Active tuberculosis**
- **Goal:** prevent treatment failure due to acquired drug resistance
- **4-drug regimen:**
- isoniazid + rifampin + pyrazinamide + ethambutol
- monthly follow-up sputum cultures
- patient compliance is most important!

*Previous BCG vaccination produces skin reactivity, but induration >15mm should be considered positive.*

# 3.265.) TULAREMIA

= rabbit fever, extremely rare in US now

| Risk factors | **reservoir:** white rabbits, rodents…<br>**vectors:** ticks, fleas… |
|---|---|
| Prevention | • tick repellents<br>• avoid contact with rabbits and rodents |
| Management | ➤ streptomycin |


# 3.266.) TURNER'S SYNDROME

| Prevention | • prenatal detection for couples with chromosome translocations |
|---|---|
| Management | **Genetic counseling:**<br>• low fertility rate<br>• if pregnant: high risk of chromosomal abnormalities in offspring |

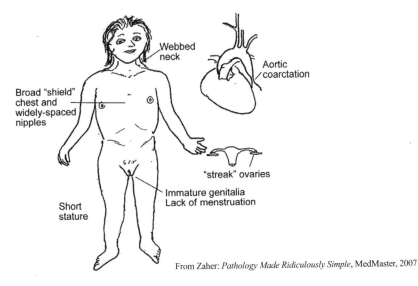

Webbed neck

Aortic coarctation

Broad "shield" chest and widely-spaced nipples

"streak" ovaries

Immature genitalia
Lack of menstruation

Short stature

From Zaher: *Pathology Made Ridiculously Simple*, MedMaster, 2007

# 3.267.) TYPHOID FEVER

S. typhi - S. paratyphi A and B - S. typhimurium

| | |
|---|---|
| **Risk factors** | o travel to tropical countries<br>o contaminated water<br>o human carriers |
| **Prevention** | • avoid tap water<br>• avoid salads, raw vegetables<br>• avoid unpeeled fruits<br>➢ vaccine if traveling to high-risk endemic area |
| **Management** | ➢ ciprofloxacin or 3$^{rd}$ generation cephalosporin<br>• cholecystectomy if relapsing |

*Non-typhoid salmonellosis is much more common in US than typhoid fever.*

# 3.268.) TYPHUS FEVER

| | |
|---|---|
| **Risk factors** | **RESERVOIR**    **VECTOR** |
| | epidemic typhus:       humans      lice <br> scrub typhus:          rodents      mites <br> endemic (murine) typhus:  rodents      fleas |
| **Prevention** | • sanitation <br> • avoid vectors |
| **Management** | ➢ all *Rickettsia* are sensitive to tetracycline |
| **Prognosis** | epidemic typhus:   50% mortality untreated <br> scrub typhus:     30% mortality untreated <br> endemic typhus:   < 2% mortality untreated |

# 3.269.) ULCERATIVE COLITIS

**Risk factors**

- o Caucasians
- o Jews
- o family history
- o major psychological stress → trigger

**Prognosis**

75% will relapse
20% will require colectomy

---

**1. Diet during flare-ups**
- high-protein
- low-fiber

↓

**2. Medical therapy**
- sulfasalazine (5-ASA is the active moiety)
- if unresponsive: oral glucocorticoids
  immuno-modulators
- acute and severe colitis: IV glucocorticoids

↓

**3. Surgical therapy**
Indications:
- colitis unresponsive to medical therapy
- toxic megacolon unresponsive to antibiotics

✓ Surgery is curative, but rarely needed

---

*Colonoscopy should be performed every 1~2 years to detect dysplasia or colon cancer. If high-grade dysplasia, consider colectomy.*

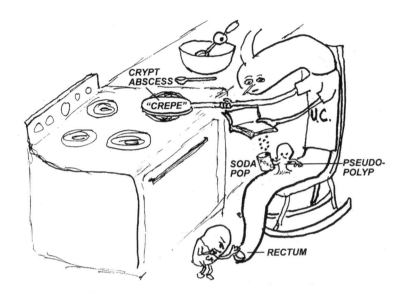

From Zaher: *Pathology Made Ridiculously Simple*, MedMaster, 2007

# 3.270.) <u>URINARY INCONTINENCE</u>

| | |
|---|---|
| **Risk factors** | o age<br>o multiparity<br>o diabetes |
| **Prevention** | • Kegel exercises after child birth |
| **Management** | **1.** exclude UTI<br>**2.** pelvic muscle exercises<br>**3.** anticholinergic drugs<br>**4.** consider surgery for stress incontinence |

# 3.271.) URINARY TRACT INFECTION

| | |
|---|---|
| **Risk factors** | o  diabetes mellitus<br>o  pregnancy<br>o  prostate hypertrophy<br>o  sexual activity<br>o  catheter use |
| **Prevention** | •  maintain good hydration<br>•  sparse use of catheters |
| **Management** | **Empirical antibiotics:**<br>➢  trimethoprim-sulfamethoxazole<br>➢  fluoroquinolone<br><br>•  if signs of pyelonephritis: get urine culture before starting antibiotics |

# 3.272.) UTERINE MYOMAS

| | |
|---|---|
| **Prevalence** | 40% of women > 50 years,  most are asymptomatic |
| **Risk factors** | o  African Americans |
| **Management** | **1.** exclude pregnancy – then get endometrial biopsy<br>**2.** if asymptomatic: no treatment necessary<br>**3.** if mild symptoms: oral contraceptives or progesterone<br>**4.** if severe symptoms: myomectomy or hysterectomy |
| **Prognosis** | •  usually decrease in size after menopause<br>•  10% recurrence following myomectomy |

 *Caution: may mask other (potentially lethal) pelvic tumors.*

# 3.273.) VAGINAL CANCER

| | |
|---|---|
| **Risk factors** | **Squamous carcinoma**<br>○ HPV<br>○ smoking<br><br>**Clear cell carcinoma**<br>○ daughters of mothers who took DES [1] |
| **Prevention** | • annual Pap smear |
| **Management** | **1.** radiation<br>**2.** if localized to upper 1/3: radical hysterectomy with upper vaginectomy |
| **Prognosis** | <u>**5-year survival**</u><br><br>**Stage I** (limited to mucosa)        - 80%<br>**Stage II** (invades subvaginal tissue)  - 60%<br>**Stage III** (extends to pelvic wall)    - 40%<br>**Stage IV** (invades rectum or bladder) - 10% |

[1] *up to 0.1% of exposed female fetuses*

## 3.274.) VENTRICULAR SEPTAL DEFECT
most common congenital heart defect

| | |
|---|---|
| **Risk factors** | o increased risk if sibling affected |
| **Prevention** | • for adults: reduce risk factors for MI |
| **Management** | 1. small defects may be left unrepaired.<br>2. surgical closure should be performed before pulmonary hypertension develops!<br>3. if pulmonary vascular disease develops, heart-lung transplant becomes the only option. |
| **Prognosis** | **congenital:** 50% will close spontaneously |

## 3.275.) VITILIGO
loss of melanin pigment

| | |
|---|---|
| **Risk factors** | o family history in 30%<br>o often triggered by stressful event |
| **Management** | 1. PUVA: psoralen plus UV light<br>2. topical glucocorticoids may help repigmentation<br>3. avoid sun exposure while treated! |

 *Search for thyroid or autoimmune disease.*

# 3.276.) WARTS
### verruca vulgaris

| | |
|---|---|
| **Risk factors** | o immunosuppression<br>o atopic dermatitis<br>o locker rooms |
| **Prevention** | • avoid wound fluid after cryotherapy |
| **Management** | **1.** cryotherapy<br>**2.** keratolytics: salicylic acid plasters |
| **Prognosis** | warts often regress spontaneously |

# 3.277.) WILMS' TUMOR
### nephroblastoma

| | |
|---|---|
| **Risk factors** | o aniridia<br>o cryptorchidism<br>o hypospadia<br>o other urogenital abnormalities |
| **Management** | **1.** surgical resection<br>**2.** adjuvant chemotherapy or radiation |
| **Prognosis** | **favorable histology:** 90% survival<br>**unfavorable histology:** 50~70% survival |

*Second most common abdominal tumor in children (after neuroblastoma).*

# 3.278.) ZOLLINGER-ELLISON SYNDROME

| | |
|---|---|
| **Risk factors** | o 25% of cases with MEN 1<br>o 75% occur sporadic |
| **2° Prevention** | • screen all first degree relatives for MEN |
| **Management** | **1.** high-dose proton pump inhibitor<br><br>**2.** get CT or scintigraphy<br>  if no metastases → attempt surgical cure and<br>        duodenectomy<br>  surgery is controversial if a/w MEN1<br><br>**3.** if gastrectomy is necessary: replace B12, iron… |
| **Prognosis** | surgical cure almost 50% if <u>sporadic</u> |

*Gastrinomas arise in the pancreas or duodenum and are*
*slow growing. 2/3 are malignant → liver metastases.*

# ABBREVIATIONS

| | | | |
|---|---|---|---|
| a/w | associated with | IVP | intravenous pyelography |
| AA | amyloid A protein | LBBB | left bundle branch block |
| ACE | angiotensin converting enzyme | LDL | low density lipoproteins |
| AFP | alpha fetoprotein | LES | lower esophageal sphincter |
| AIP | acute intermittent porphyria | LFT | liver function tests |
| AJCC | Am. Joint Commission on Cancer | LMN | lower motor neuron |
| AL | amyloid light chains: κ, λ | MALT | mucosa-associated lymphoid tissue |
| ANA | antinuclear antibodies | MCHC | mean corpuscular hemoglobin |
| ANLL | acute non-lymphocytic leukemia | | concentration |
| ASD | atrial septal defect | MCV | mean corpuscular volume |
| ATN | acute tubular necrosis | MEN | multiple endocrine neoplasia |
| BCG | bacillus Calmette-Guérin | MGUS | monoclonal gammopathy of |
| BP | blood pressure | | unknown significance |
| BPH | benign prostate hyperplasia | MI | myocardial infarction |
| CDC | Center for Disease Control | MR | mitral regurgitation |
| CHF | congestive heart failure | MS | mitral stenosis |
| CMML | chronic myelomonocytic | NIDDM | non-insulin-dependent diabetes |
| | leukemia | | mellitus |
| CMV | cytomegalovirus | OSHA | Occupational Safety and Health |
| COPD | chronic obstructive pulmonary | | Administration |
| | disease | PCP | Pneumocystis pneumonia |
| COX | cyclooxygenase | PCT | porphyria cutanea tarda |
| CPK | creatine phosphokinase | PFT | pulmonary function tests |
| CVA | cerebrovascular accident | PID | pelvic inflammatory disease |
| CXR | chest X-ray | PMS | premenstrual syndrome |
| DES | diethylstilbestrol | PPD | purified protein derivative |
| DIC | disseminated intravascular | PPI | proton pump inhibitor |
| | coagulation | PSA | prostate specific antigen |
| DM | diabetes mellitus | RBBB | right bundle branch block |
| DPT | diphtheria-pertussis-tetanus | RSV | respiratory syncytial virus |
| DVT | deep vein thrombosis | SAAG | serum-ascites albumin gradient |
| EBV | Epstein-Barr virus | SBFT | small bowel follow through |
| EEE | eastern equine encephalitis | SSPE | subacute sclerosing panencephalitis |
| ENG | electronystagmography | STD | sexually transmitted disease |
| ERCP | endoscopic retrograde | TIA | transient ischemic attack |
| | cholangiopancreatography | TIBC | total iron binding capacity |
| ESR | erythrocyte sedimentation rate | TTP | thrombotic thrombocytopenic |
| FNA | fine needle aspiration | | purpura |
| GN | glomerulonephritis | tPA | tissue plasminogen activator |
| HDL | high density lipoproteins | UGI | upper gastrointestinal |
| HPV | human papilloma virus | UTI | urinary tract infection |
| IDDM | insulin-dependent diabetes mellitus | UMN | upper motor neuron |
| ITP | idiopathic thrombocytopenic | VDRL | Venereal Disease Research Lab's |
| | purpura | VSD | ventricular septal defect |
| IUD | intrauterine device | WPW | Wolff-Parkinson-White syndrome |

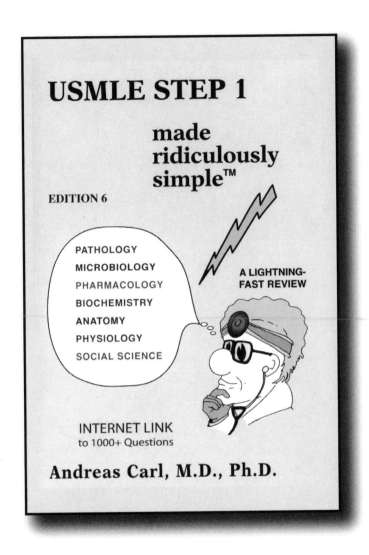

USMLE STEP 1

made
ridiculously
simple™

EDITION 6

PATHOLOGY
MICROBIOLOGY
PHARMACOLOGY
BIOCHEMISTRY
ANATOMY
PHYSIOLOGY
SOCIAL SCIENCE

A LIGHTNING-
FAST REVIEW

INTERNET LINK
to 1000+ Questions

Andreas Carl, M.D., Ph.D.

**422 pages  -  335 charts**

♦ All the Facts about Basic Medical Sciences in a Unique Chart Format.

♦ Clinical Correlations, Tips and Hints.

♦ Easy to Memorize !!!

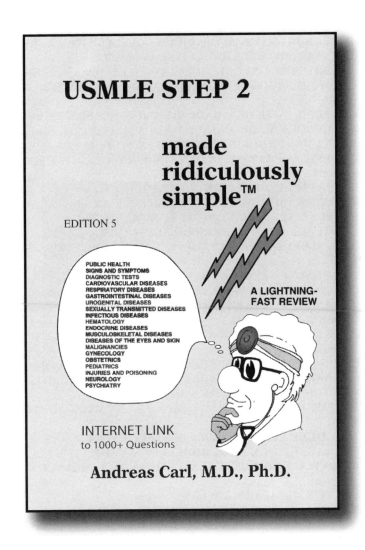

**404 pages - 280 charts**

♦ Systematic Review of Diseases and Organ Systems in Chart Format

♦ Patient Management and Therapy

♦ Easy to Memorize !!!

*RAPID LEARNING AND RETENTION THROUGH THE MEDMASTER SERIES:*

CLINICAL NEUROANATOMY MADE RIDICULOUSLY SIMPLE, by S. Goldberg
CLINICAL BIOCHEMISTRY MADE RIDICULOUSLY SIMPLE, by S. Goldberg
CLINICAL ANATOMY MADE RIDICULOUSLY SIMPLE, by S. Goldberg
CLINICAL PHYSIOLOGY MADE RIDICULOUSLY SIMPLE, by S. Goldberg
CLINICAL MICROBIOLOGY MADE RIDICULOUSLY SIMPLE, by M. Gladwin
and B. Trattler
CLINICAL PHARMACOLOGY MADE RIDICULOUSLY SIMPLE, by J.M. Olson
OPHTHALMOLOGY MADE RIDICULOUSLY SIMPLE, by S. Goldberg
PSYCHIATRY MADE RIDICULOUSLY SIMPLE, by W.V. Good and J. Nelson
CLINICAL PSYCHOPHARMACOLOGY MADE RIDICULOUSLY SIMPLE,
by J. Preston and J. Johnson
USMLE STEP 1 MADE RIDICULOUSLY SIMPLE, by A. Carl
USMLE STEP 2 MADE RIDICULOUSLY SIMPLE, by A. Carl
USMLE STEP 3 MADE RIDICULOUSLY SIMPLE, by A. Carl
BEHAVIORAL MEDICINE MADE RIDICULOUSLY SIMPLE, by F. Seitz and J. Carr
ACID-BASE, FLUIDS, AND ELECTROLYTES MADE RIDICULOUSLY SIMPLE,
by R. Preston
THE FOUR-MINUTE NEUROLOGIC EXAM, by S. Goldberg
MEDICAL SPANISH MADE RIDICULOUSLY SIMPLE, by T. Espinoza-Abrams
CLINICAL ANATOMY AND PHYSIOLOGY FOR THE ANGRY HEALTH
PROFESSIONAL, by J.V. Stewart
PREPARING FOR MEDICAL PRACTICE MADE RIDICULOUSLY SIMPLE,
by D.M. Lichtstein
MED'TOONS (260 humorous medical cartoons by the author) by S. Goldberg
CLINICAL RADIOLOGY MADE RIDICULOUSLY SIMPLE, by H. Ouellette
NCLEX-RN MADE RIDICULOUSLY SIMPLE, by A. Carl
THE PRACTITIONER'S POCKET PAL: ULTRA RAPID MEDICAL REFERENCE,
by J. Hancock
ORGANIC CHEMISTRY MADE RIDICULOUSLY SIMPLE, by G.A. Davis
CLINICAL CARDIOLOGY MADE RIDICULOUSLY SIMPLE, by M.A. Chizner
PSYCHIATRY ROUNDS: PRACTICAL SOLUTIONS TO CLINICAL CHALLENGES,
by N.A. Vaidya and M.A. Taylor.
MEDMASTER'S MEDSEARCHER, by S. Goldberg
PATHOLOGY MADE RIDICULOUSLY SIMPLE, by A. Zaher
CLINICAL PATHOPHYSIOLOGY MADE RIDICULOUSLY SIMPLE, by A. Berkowitz
ATLAS OF MICROBIOLOGY, by S. Goldberg
ATLAS OF DERMATOLOGY, by S. Goldberg and B. Galitzer
ATLAS OF HUMAN DISEASES, by S. Goldberg
ORTHOPEDICS MADE RIDICULOUSLY SIMPLE, by P. Tétreault and H. Ouellette
ATLAS OF ORTHOPEDICS, by P. Tétreault, H. Ouellette, and S. Goldberg
ANATOMY OF THE SOUL, by S. Goldberg
IMMUNOLOGY MADE RIDICULOUSLY SIMPLE, by M. Mahmoudi
CLINICAL BIOSTATISTICS MADE RIDICULOUSLY SIMPLE, by A. Weaver
and S. Goldberg

Try your bookstore. For further information and ordering send for the MedMaster catalog
at MedMaster, P.O. Box 640028, Miami FL 33164. Or see http://www.medmaster.net for
current information. Email: mmbks@aol.com.